I0102507

www.facilitatingbalance.com

Images: www.horstfriedrichs.com
Cover design: 1/2 Full Studios

ISBN 978-0-9956802-2-7

Copyright © 2016 Facilitating Balance

Contents

Introduction

Today's lifestyle often involves juggling work and home lives, battling deadlines, toiling in artificial environments, enduring long hours commuting, eating hurriedly as well as being bombarded by sounds, images and pollutants. It is not surprising that stress levels, depression and anxiety along with numerous stress related physical problems seem to be on the increase.

Many of us have developed our own ways of trying to maintain a balanced state, perhaps by exercising, or by having an enjoyable hobby or healthy loving relationships, all of which help us to wind down and relax. Sometimes we use alcohol, drugs or other less constructive methods. We all appear to have a drive to find a sense of balance, even if we do not always choose the right road to get there.

Whilst it is not always possible to improve one's immediate environment, by learning a few simple tools and putting certain routines in place, we can gain a sense of perspective and control which hopefully minimises the negative physical and emotional impacts of our stressful lives.

There are different tools to achieve this end and we cannot include them all in this book. However we hope that the reader will be able to relate to their own experiences in making use of some of the strategies described here, to help facilitate a sense of balance.

Wherever possible, scientific explanations and details are provided. For those unfamiliar with some of the terminology, it is hoped the basic concepts will still be accessible and practical. The areas explored include:

- The influence of stress and thinking on heart function and our ability to make rational objective decisions.

- Processing of emotive events by the mind and enhancing mindfulness through meditation.

- How natural cycles in the day affect concentration and healing.

- Food and its effect on brain chemistry and mood.

- Ayurvedic complementary concepts; looking at how lifestyles, seasons and foods may affect us as individuals.

- Taking breaks.

- Therapeutic use of light in helping mood and levels of alertness.

- Use of food supplements and herbal remedies.

- Dietary intake of omega-3 fatty acids.

- Alcohol use and resources.

- Drug use and resources.

- Conflict resolution.

- Sleep hygiene.

What Is Stress?

Stress may be regarded as any taxation on our being, be it physical, mental or both, that uses up our resources. It may be positive when exercising hard or staying up late with a group of friends and having an enjoyable time. Such experiences can be beneficial through the psychological and physical reinforcement they provide.

Stress may be negative when dealing with a difficult boss, not having time to eat or sleep properly due to obligations to others, or having to deal with major events in life such as bereavement. These situations may be accompanied by a sense of entrapment and result in unhealthy physiological and psychological effects, the opposite of the positive reinforcement that comes from stresses that we enjoy.

It should be noted that even enjoyable stresses can be detrimental, if they involve abuse of our normal sleep cycle, brain chemistry or the body itself.

Signs of stress may vary from person to person and if ongoing may result in: periods of sickness, fatigue, mistakes, strained relationships, a decrease in creativity and productivity, a sense of resentment, irritability, frustration, anxiety or depression.

It Goes Through The Heart

When we experience negative emotions, such as irritation, anger, anxiety or sadness, the body reacts by increasing blood pressure and releasing the stress hormone cortisol. There is also a drop in type A immunoglobulin (Ig.A) antibodies for some hours(1). These antibodies are found in the mucosal lining of our nose, throat, lungs, intestines and form part of the body's immune system.

Another response is a decrease in heart rate variability, a natural phenomenon of the heart. These negative physical changes result in decreased functioning of the logical part of the brain (the neocortex) making it more difficult to maintain perspective, work efficiently and make objective decisions.

The opposite also occurs: a positive thought will have a positive effect, increasing our heart rate variability and our Ig.A levels, as well as allowing us to work with a sense of perspective.

Heart rate variability is our heart's natural ability to gently increase and decrease its rate in response to a balanced working of the two parts of our nervous system, the parasympathetic slowing the body down and the sympathetic speeding it up. Poor heart rate variability is now recognised as a good predictor of death due to progressive heart failure or following a myocardial infarct.

Imbalance in an overactive sympathetic system due to stress will reduce heart rate variability and make it difficult to maintain full functioning of our neocortex, the "logical brain".

This may be useful if we have to react quickly to a physical threat, such as moving out the way of a vehicle without thinking, which helps to save valuable time. It is less useful if trying to function in an office environment, where an agitated physical and emotional state can hinder us from making appropriate decisions. Often there is no physical release for the body, now alerted to physically react to a stressful situation with what is known as "a fight or flight response", a survival instinct that would have primed us to fight or run from a predator.

When the two systems are in balance and heart rate variability is good, this state is called cardiac coherence. When not in balance, it is known as cardiac chaos. People may not be aware that their heart rate variability has become chaotic as it may not be accompanied by any strongly felt physical change. However measurement of variability can show how it can easily shift, stirred even by angry or pleasant thoughts.

Regular coherence states can result in decreased levels of the stress hormone cortisol, associated with skin ageing, loss of memory and increased blood pressure(2). Coherence will help to increase DHEA (dehydroepiandrosterone)(3), a hormone that is associated with a reduction in blood pressure(4). The ratio of cortisol to DHEA usually increases with age and may mean a less effective immune system(5). Coherence can help to reduce this change.

In coherence it is easier to get on with day to day functioning because less physical and emotional energy is required. It also helps to maintain a healthy immune system. Some of us have learnt to stay close to such a state, perhaps by recalling a happy memory or a loved one, or having a family photo on our phone or desk. Others may use prayer or meditative techniques, or even take a few deep sighs at times of duress.

If you find yourself feeling a warm glow after a pleasant event or at the recollection of a pleasant memory, you are likely to be in a state of coherence. When breathing out deeply, as in a sigh, we automatically stimulate our parasympathetic system, slowing the heart down and dampening the sympathetic system. Such breathing techniques are consciously employed in such practices as Pilates or yoga.

To practise regaining coherence through breathing, we can:

- Find a quiet place to sit for about 15 to 20 minutes. Lie down if unable to sit.

- Breathe normally and just relax for a few moments.

- Take your attention to the centre of your chest and imagine your breath coming into the body through the heart and then going out through the heart. If you like, you can think of the breath as a rejuvenating white light.

- Breathe naturally so the body can relax into a nice deep pattern of breathing. You should find there is a few seconds pause between the end of the out breath and starting to inhale again.

- Whilst doing this try to maintain a positive thought, image or pleasant memory that makes you feel good.

As your awareness of your breath increases, this will become easier and you will be able to establish coherence by the breath technique, or even by imagining a positive image or scenario. In fact I suggest you have a few of these ready for stressful occasions and don't be afraid to practise the breath technique just before and after a difficult encounter. Try to ground yourself if feeling the need to react, before going on to do something else. If you find yourself really upset by something, make use of the strategies explored later to influence mood with food.

Coherence should become easier with time and increased awareness. The breath focused mindful meditation described later should also help to enhance your ability to achieve coherence. There are computer programmes and hand held biofeedback devices that can help to monitor and promote a coherent state. These are available through Heart Math, via Hunter Kane in the UK. They may be found at www.hunterkane.com

Emotional Trauma

Earlier we mentioned the need for survival instincts, which originate in an area of the brain called the amygdala. This area is associated with emotions and it both influences and is influenced by heart rate, relationships, sleep cycle and sensory stimuli. We can act on this part of the brain through the body, for example through coherence and meditative techniques, massage, eye movements, or acupressure.

Alone, the emotional brain is not able to engage appropriately with the world. For this we need the neocortex, our logical brain, to inhibit certain impulses and allow us to regulate our behaviour within the cultural and social norms we experience. It is also required to give us the attention and concentration we need for complex tasks.

When these two parts of the brain are working in harmony, we are able to function well, work logically, perceive danger appropriately and make objective decisions.

In certain situations where the emotional brain has become overactive, logical reasoning is lost. It may be submerged for a short while, perhaps in the heat of argument where there is physical agitation. But it can become a longer term problem, for example in post traumatic stress disorder, where a powerful experience such as a mugging, torture or car accident may have left us with an unresolved emotional memory that we have not "processed".

Dealing with such experiences can be difficult and at times require professional input and even medication to get close enough to the experience to "process" it, in order to let go of it. This "processing" can only happen in the absence of severe physical agitation.

Ignoring such emotional pain, using logical justification or looking for escape in drugs, alcohol or self-destructive behaviour only increases the impact of such memories on the mind and body. This may then manifest itself in different ways for different people:

through hypertension, decreased immunity, gastrointestinal or skin problems, depressive features or anxiety.

Whilst a direct correlation can sometimes be difficult to establish in a measured scientific way, there is an increasing appreciation of the impact of emotive experiences on both mental and physical health. Depression, where mental and physical manifestations of stressful life events can occur, is a good example of this.

The mind does not like to leave such emotional memories alone. It will keep going over them, in order to "process" them, so we can slowly let them go. We can probably all recall an experience, such as an argument with a close friend, where afterwards we kept going over it in our mind, until it became less intense. The gradual reduction in physical agitation accompanying such recollection helps us to let go.

Really powerful traumas are very hard to deal with, as every time the mind recalls them our body reacts by getting agitated, our heart rate and blood pressure rising as a result of an overactive sympathetic system, causing cardiac chaos. This in turn inhibits our neocortex, the logical part of the brain.

We need our neocortex to be functioning well in order to process these traumas so that we can begin to let them go. When our neocortex is shut down, the traumatic memories will keep coming back. If we consciously try to suppress such memories they may well come back in our sleep and if we are made physically uncomfortable by a strong sympathetic response, we may well be awoken from sleep.

This can result in a vicious cycle of repeated painful memories, physical agitation and disruption of sleep, all resulting in avoidance and suppression with long term mental and physical consequences.

There is no emotional processing without a functioning neocortex and therefore a relaxed physical state. Some people are so traumatised that they may require a combination of antipsychotic and antidepressant medication to help them sleep and to dampen their overactive sympathetic system and traumatic memories.

Other people may be able to manage this emotional processing through therapies, where the body is distracted from the painful memory by another activity which dampens down the sympathetic response. Examples of this might be:

- Talking to a therapist.

- Drawing pictures as representations of the event.

- Writing about the event.

- Using eye movement desensitisation reprocessing, known as EMDR, a technique where eye movements are directed from one side to the other, whilst the memory is accessed.

- Using mindful meditation techniques.

In my experience with severely traumatised patients, initially medication and then later use of other techniques may be required. The extremely agitated physical state needs time to settle and any premature conscious recall of the event worsens the agitation.

As mentioned earlier "logical" reasoning alone is not enough. Logically understanding an emotional event and emotionally making peace with it are two different things. We might understand why a loved one may have over-reacted towards us in a negative way, but coming to terms with that emotionally is something else. The same applies if one is mugged, attacked or the victim of an earthquake.

In the next section we look at one of the therapeutic tools referred to above, to allow for greater neocortical processing, that is, mindful meditation. Like cardiac coherence, once learnt, it is easy to practise on one's own and can be a very powerful tool for maintaining coherence and objectivity, as well as acting as a catalyst for our development.

For those dealing with very traumatic events, professional therapeutic input and medication may also have a strong role to play. For such people I suggest supervised meditation to begin with.

Mindful Meditation

Studies have shown a number benefits from mindful meditation. These have included lowering of blood pressure and decreased insulin resistance(1), where the latter usually increases in diabetes. There have also been improved symptoms of post traumatic stress disorder as well as electroencepholograph (EEG) coherence(2). EEG represents a recording of brain activity, with coherence indicating good levels of alertness and concentration.

Other studies have shown a decrease in stress and supporting of forgiveness(3), enhanced coping and well being in cancer patients(4), and decreased seizure frequency and duration in drug resistant epileptics(5). Long-standing practitioners have shown evidence of increased cortical thickening (outer tissue of the brain) on magnetic resonance imaging (MRI) scanning, in the frontal cortex and right anterior insula areas of the brain(6).

Meditation works on three main levels. The first involves getting the body into a very relaxed state, where your blood pressure and pulse may drop, with breathing slowing into a deep rhythmic pattern. When your body is in this state, it is easier for the mind to process any emotive material it needs to – the second level. This is only possible if there is a settled physiological state when getting close to memories or emotions.

The third aspect is practising what is called mindfulness. This is a state of awareness where one observes one's thoughts, emotions, physical state and surroundings, being in the moment, not judging or reacting to things, rather acknowledging what is present. This can help in maintaining a broad perspective and, if required, taking appropriate action.

A simple example of this would be walking down the street and having someone shout aggressively at you for no good reason. Your initial reaction may be fear, irritation or anger - an emotional response. Mindfulness would enable you to acknowledge the feelings present and allow you to take a conscious course of action, rather than just being reactive. This could be to ignore them, walk away, try to reason with them or even come to the realisation that they may be mentally unwell. Any of these may be possible if there is not a strong emotional outburst leaving you no option of choice. Learning to be less physiologically reactive aids mindfulness and gives you this opportunity to exercise choice.

By staying in the moment, mindfulness allows us to acknowledge our own responses to emotional events and memories from a healthier perspective, rather than be carried away by them. It should help facilitate a sense of awareness and honesty, enabling us to take responsibility when required, rather than blame others. It can help us to challenge negative patterns of thinking and promote change towards more constructive decision-making and behaviour.

Mindfulness may be easier to practise when meditating, but can be practised at any time, by using tools that bring you back to the moment. This could be by becoming aware of your breath, which is always in the present, or aware of your feet touching the pavement when walking, or completely connecting with an activity. A good example is the Japanese tea ceremony, where the whole experience involves an attentiveness to every detail, from boiling water, to the texture of the cup, to the taste of the tea. In fact, any activity you engage in can be done mindfully, by connecting with it fully.

A very simple way of practising mindfulness is to slow down whatever you are doing - walking, talking or eating for example. You may find it a very useful tool for regaining a sense of perspective and being able to connect more fully with any activity you engage in.

There are different ways to meditate. Most people use a focal point, like the breath, a word (mantra) that you keep coming back to, or a visual image. We will look at a simple breath focused technique.

Meditating twice a day for 20 minutes, anywhere you feel comfortable, is good practice. This could be in the morning, before tea, coffee or breakfast. You may have a glass of juice or freshen up first. If you have no option but to eat or have tea or coffee, you can still meditate afterwards.

The afternoon or early evening, when you are returning home from work, maybe on public transport, or when you arrive home, ideally before tea or coffee, is a suitable time for your second meditation. The morning meditation acts as a good buffer for the day and the evening helps to process the day. It should be noted that our natural rhythm is to begin slowing down from about 4pm. Meditating close to this time can benefit us greatly.

Try to avoid meditating late at night. Whilst you will be physically relaxed, you may become mentally alert, making it difficult to fall asleep soon after. This is especially the case if you have come out of the meditative state fully: if not, you may be able to sleep without difficulty by allowing yourself to lie down during the process.

There will be more about coming out of the meditation later.

The Procedure

Sit in a comfortable position with your back straight and well supported but make sure your head is not resting back, as you don't just want to relax and fall asleep - remember we are also practising mindfulness. Try to keep your head and back straight. It is fine to sit in a chair or on the floor - as you like. It could be anywhere you feel comfortable, inside or outside. If you are unable to sit you may lie down.

We can use a simple body awareness technique to prepare for the meditation. Start by closing your eyes and becoming aware of your feet, allowing yourself to simply feel them there, then your lower legs, followed by your upper legs, next your abdomen, chest, shoulders, upper arms, lower arms, hands, neck, head and face.

We now start becoming aware of our breath, breathing normally. Observe your breath, the sensation and sound of air flowing in and out of your nostrils, into your chest. You will find your mind wandering to other things, maybe noises around you, or some thoughts or feelings. When this happens just acknowledge whatever your mind is doing and come back to the breath. Soon your mind will wander again; just acknowledge it and come back to the breath.

It is normal for the mind to wander, as it is its nature. Do not be upset or too forceful when this occurs: return gently to the breath, which acts like an anchor.

After five to ten minutes of this, you will begin to go into the meditative state, with the physiological changes mentioned. You may find your mind becoming very active, processing things it needs to. There should be a sense of watching your mind do this, like being in a train and seeing things go by in the window. You should have a sense of being still; even though your mind may be busy with imagery, that is your sense of mindfulness.

Don't worry too much about what you see or what it means. Some things will be obvious, but a lot may be happening at a deeper subconscious level. It is impossible to fathom what is at the bottom of a lake from the ripples on the surface. The main thing is the process and emotionally making peace with things that are concerning you. Remember to have your breath in the background. It is your anchor and always in the present, regardless of where your mind may be.

Every meditation you practise will be different. After a good sleep your mind may be very quiet, after work it may take longer to settle down. Your meditation will continue to change with practice. Don't worry if you don't always get into a really relaxed state, as this is being mindful of comfort and discomfort.

When meditating, you may become aware of tension in different parts of the body. We all store stress in different ways; if you have any discomfort, go there with your mind, connect with it, keeping the awareness of your breath in the background. You should find that the tension dissipates, through muscle contractions in the area or even tears. It will be different for everyone, but the main rule is not to fight it, but to take your awareness there without being forceful.

When you start meditating you can keep time by setting an alarm or glancing at a watch during the meditation; gradually you will become accustomed to the passage of time. Ideally, you should plan not to be interrupted. However, if you have no choice but to open the door or answer the phone, do so and then go back to your meditation.

Ending The Meditation

It is important not to rush when finishing your meditation, as this can give you a headache. If this happens, go back, let things settle and come out slowly. To help you come out of the meditative state, you can turn your attention to sounds around you, take a few deep breaths, in through the nose and out through the mouth, stretch your arms and legs and keeping your gaze down, slowly allow light to enter your eyes. Allow yourself a few minutes to do all this.

During this time, you may want to practise the cardiac coherence exercise for a few minutes. Alternatively, you may use this time to visualise a positive outcome for a problem or difficult task you face.

Afterwards, resting for ten to 15 minutes will help you maintain this state for longer. Perhaps you can use the time to eat. If you are physically ill, you can meditate as much as you want to. If there is deep emotive material being processed, it may take time to work through and on occasion can leave you feeling physically drained, sometimes for days. If this happens make sure you get plenty of rest.

The main thing to remember is to keep things simple, use your breath as your anchor, don't force anything, let things come and go. We don't have to hang on to them. If they come back, let them come and then let them go again. Sometimes the mind has to go over things again and again in order to make peace with them. This is its way of processing emotional material. So long as you are in a physically relaxed state during these times, there should be progress.

Try to think of mindfulness at other times, practise it as much as possible, whatever you are doing. It will get easier and easier and allow you the awareness to acknowledge what is present, accept it or if required challenge it; whether it is a feeling you haven't come to terms with or a pattern of thinking that doesn't serve a useful purpose. At such times you may want to ask yourself what are the benefits of holding on to a way of thinking and if this might be improved upon to support you better.

Always treat yourself as you would a child. Criticism should be constructive, supportive and always accompanied with love. Accept and acknowledge whatever is there with love and then choose where you want to go. Try not to get upset because things are not as you wish, or because you are unable to change things quickly. It is a process.

Your freedom lies in choosing your actions and not in being able to determine all aspects of your life, which are guaranteed to change and are often outside your control. With time and increased mindfulness, your ability to develop will continue to improve.

Take a look at the meditation organisation site www.vipassana.org - they have a book on their site called Mindfulness in Plain English by Venerable Henepola Gunaratana, which may help you to understand this concept and meditation more easily. It can also be ordered through bookshops.

Meditation Summary

Introduction

- A tool for relaxation and working through stresses.
- Can be practised anywhere you feel comfortable.
- Ideally for 20 minutes twice a day, preferably before breakfast, tea or coffee and early evening before dinner.
- Meditating before sleeping may make you feel more alert, unless you do not come out of your meditation and allow yourself to fall asleep.
- It is a different state to sleeping, dreaming or being awake.
- The body's physiology is different in this state, with a drop in blood pressure and respiratory rate and increased cardiac coherence.
- The longer you experience meditation, the more your ability to maintain this state will improve.

Procedure

- There are different ways of meditating.
- Most use a focal point for their awareness; this can be a sound (word), visual image or the breath.
- It is not about forcing the mind into stillness: it is more likely to become still when it has worked through certain stresses.
- This technique uses body awareness (feet, calves, thighs, abdomen, chest, shoulders, upper arms, lower arms, neck, head, face) followed by focusing on the breath.
- Focusing on the breath is a tool to get you into a meditative state and aids you in maintaining mindfulness.
- Your mind will drift to other thoughts; let these thoughts finish then come back to your breath.
- It is not necessary to force things or be upset if you cannot easily stay with your breath, just keep gently coming back to it.

What is experienced?

- Every meditation is different, depending on your state.
- Common themes may be an increase in imagery or thoughts (the train window analogy), before your mind becomes quiet.
- The imagery is in itself unimportant (the lake analogy).
- Towards the later stages you may experience a calm state of awareness, or during the meditation drift in and out of calm periods.
- Sometimes you may experience tension in parts of the body, if this happens, allow your awareness to go there, it usually helps to relieve it.

Ending the meditation

- After 20 minutes (you can look at your watch to check the time) take a few deep breaths, stretch your arms and legs and open your eyes slowly. This should help you to come out of the meditation.
- You may want to practise the cardiac coherence technique for a few minutes, breathing "through the heart" to help reinforce this practice at other times, or visualise a positive outcome for a task or situation.
- Take a few minutes before you start to do other things.
- Rushing can give you a headache. If this seems imminent allow yourself to go back into the meditation, let things settle and then come out slowly.
- Resting for 10 - 15 minutes afterwards can be quite beneficial.

Guided Meditation Audio Download

Available at www.facilitatingbalance.com/meditation

Dancing To The Ultradian Rhythm

Here we will take a look at why spending at least two sessions a day on activities that promote states such as cardiac coherence through relaxation or meditation supports our natural make-up.

We are all aware of different rhythms and cycles governing our lives, day to night, menstrual, seasonal and lunar to name a few. There are also the circadian (24 hour) cycles which affect the release of hormones. Men's testosterone levels, for example, peaking in the morning whilst the release of growth hormone occurs during sleep at around 2am.

The circadian cycle also causes a gradual peaking of our levels of alertness from waking onwards. Then there is a shifting to a slower, less active state from about 4pm, allowing us gradually to wind down and later become ready for sleep.

There are also ultradian rhythms lasting less than 24 hours which repeat many times in a day. One such ultradian cycle lasts 90 to 120 minutes and is characterised by peaking levels of alertness, with an increased ability to do complex tasks requiring intense concentration, followed by a 20 minute period where it becomes increasingly difficult to stay focused. This 20 minute period may be noticeable for:

- increased restlessness
- irritation
- wanting to pass water
- wanting to stretch or walk around
- increased desire for a snack
- difficulty staying focused on a task and making mistakes
- daydreaming
- becoming more introspective
- more frequent sexual thoughts

Our capacity for physical activity, mental alertness, hand-eye coordination and memory recall all follow this 90-120 minute cycle. This is known as the basic rest activity cycle (BRAC).

In those 20 minutes, both the mind and body are geared towards rest and replenishment, processing what we have been involved with, accessing emotions and deeper thoughts as well as connecting with our creative potential. We may also find our mind throwing up solutions to problems we have been thinking about.

Oxidative waste products and free radicals are removed and chemical molecules known as messenger molecules are replenished, these being crucial for a wide range of processes in the mind and body.

The US army department of behavioural biology at the Walter Reed Institute Of Research, Washington, found that taking 20 minute breaks every 90 minutes results in a decrease in errors, accidents and stress related disorders.

We can help support this state by taking time out, practising cardiac coherence, meditating, giving ourselves the time to leisurely move around, maybe sit on a park bench or even daydream. If feeling hungry, we can have a light snack. Ideally we should be able to attain a state of deep rhythmic breathing and cardiac coherence to maximise the nourishment of mind and body.

If we are not able to take a proper break, we can attempt a less demanding task or a different form of activity to that in which we have been engaged. If you have been sitting at a desk, move around. If you have been physically active, try something less taxing.

The work environment with its stresses and deadlines can sometimes make it difficult to register the shift into the 20 minute period, especially if we are engrossed in demanding work. However working through such cycles may make the cues such as increased restlessness harder to ignore.

Working through the 20 minute cycles with the help of stress hormones like adrenaline or stimulants like caffeine can initially give us a "rush" because of their combined impact. Over an extended period however, we can end up feeding off a cycle of highs and lows which push us towards seeking further means of achieving the high states, through increasing use of stimulants.

Ignoring our need for these breaks will mean we become less efficient, with an increase in stress levels, blood pressure, reduced cardiac coherence, immunity and self-esteem. We can also develop sleep, gastrointestinal and heart problems as well as mood disorders.

Ideally one should have at least two proper 20 minute breaks during the day, coinciding with the 20 minute slow period. An ideal time for one break, would be around 4pm or as soon as we get back from work. This will coincide with our natural disposition to slow down due to our circadian rhythm slowly preparing us for sleep.

The body's immune, endocrine and autonomic nervous systems all exhibit this 90-120 minute cycle. The stomach also contracts rhythmically every 90-120 minutes. After a meal blood sugar and insulin levels tend to peak in 90-120 minute cycles. This may cause some people to become a little hungry every 90-120 minutes. They may benefit from a small snack, ideally something such as fruit that will not cause a huge surge in blood sugar. People prone to overeating at standard mealtimes may also benefit from regular small meals at these times, to help control food intake.

Throughout our lives the timetable for the ultradian rhythm may vary. Take pregnancy - in the first trimester the foetus shares the cycle with the mother, developing its own rhythm in the second trimester. The mother may need to take longer breaks than the 20 minutes, to compensate for the increased demands on her body and to minimise production of stress hormones that can cross the placenta.

After birth, the baby's rhythm takes the form of a 40-60 minute cycle, so it may take some while for the baby's rhythm to synchronise with the mother's. At about eight months, it increases to 90-120 minute cycles. Picking up on the baby's rhythm will allow the mother gradually to synchronise with it. This will involve increased stimulation such as touching, stroking and exposure to music and light at the baby's peaking levels of alertness, but reducing this and encouraging feeding when levels of alertness fall.

It should be noted that teenage years are characterised by changing rhythms and whilst this is happening, there may be less synchronicity with other family members. At such times an understanding flexible approach may help. Older people may need more frequent breaks and should not be afraid to take them. They may find a nap of about one hour during the day can help boost growth hormone release, which aids rejuvenation and energy levels.

A similar approach can be utilised when spending time with family or friends when an appreciation of their ultradian rhythms allow you to synchronise with theirs. Joint activities such as sharing a meal, reading together or engaging in play may help. It may require about 20 minutes together to begin synchronising.

Sharing a longer period of time such as relaxing holidays without outside pressures and deadlines may allow for greater synchronisation and help in developing a sense of closeness.

Having an appreciation of our own and others' cycles can help with interactions and communication. Appreciating when people may need a little more time for self reflection or reassurance and when to make more demands on them, will all help in creating greater harmony.

Key Points

- Become aware of your rhythm and if at all possible take 20 minute breaks every 90-120 minutes.

- If you cannot take a break, change your activity to a less taxing one.

- Make use of meditation and cardiac coherence techniques to get into a deep relaxed breathing pattern for at least two 20 minute cycles.

- Do your most demanding work when your attention levels are peaking.

- Try to take a longer break for lunch; at least an hour if possible and get out of the work environment. The effect of blood being directed to your gastrointestinal system may well slow you down, making you less productive. It's a good time for a restful break.

- Look out for a larger dip in performance around late afternoon, as your circadian rhythm shifts towards slowing you down. Take a break and / or do less taxing work.

- Be mindful of the rhythms of others and appreciate that they may not be in tune with yours. It may take up to 20 minutes of shared activity to start synchronising.

- Spend regular quiet time with loved ones to help synchronise rhythms.

Maybe It's Something I Ate

So far we have explored cardiac coherence, unresolved emotional issues and cycles of alertness. Let us now take a look at the effect of food. Our brain makes use of a number of neurotransmitters that can have different effects and can also be influenced by what we eat. Here we will look at three.

Dopamine and noradrenaline are two stimulating neurotransmitters that make us feel more alert and focused. In excess they may make us feel restless, agitated or anxious. Nicotine, caffeine and other stimulants can increase their active levels. They may also be influenced by what we eat.

The precursor to these two neurotransmitters is an amino acid called tyrosine, found in protein. Providing levels in the brain are not saturated, tyrosine is taken up by the brain to form dopamine and noradrenaline. So eating a lean form of protein will, after a few hours, help to saturate the dopamine and noradrenaline levels in the brain, helping to keep us alert.

For this effect to be maximised, we need to eat about 80 gm of protein that is low in fat and eat very little carbohydrate, ideally after the protein.

People may think that ingesting something sweet that causes an increase in blood sugar would make them more alert. However this is not always the case because of the effects of insulin. Insulin is released in response to a rise in blood glucose and this release results in saturation of the third neurotransmitter we are going to look at, serotonin.

Serotonin can have a calming effect on the brain and is affected by modern antidepressants such as Prozac, which act to increase active levels in the brain. Serotonin is also involved in preparing us for sleep. Ever wondered why that big pasta meal, portion of chips, slice of cake or sweet drink made you feel too comfortable to work? Or why some colleagues may fall asleep after lunch? Chances are you were probably saturating your serotonin levels and with a large meal, diverting a lot of blood to your gastrointestinal system, all of which combine to slow you down.

Serotonin is also made from an amino acid, called tryptophan. Eating protein will increase the mount of tryptophan and tyrosine in the blood. However, when in the blood, the tryptophan is bound to a large protein molecule called albumin, which means there is less actively available to enter the brain, as albumin is not able to enter brain tissue.

There are also only so many "gates" through which these proteins enter the brain and they must compete with one another to get through. If there is more active tyrosine available, it will enter in larger amounts and cause a bigger effect by saturating noradrenaline and dopamine levels, making us feel more alert.

So how does insulin change this balance? Insulin promotes the uptake of not only sugar, but also amino acids from the blood into the tissues. This causes levels of tyrosine to fall, but as tryptophan is mostly bound to albumin, it stays in the blood. The resulting effect is that blood concentrations of free tryptophan increase. As more tryptophan is now able to pass through the "gates" with the reduced competition, more is available to the brain, saturating levels of serotonin and making you more relaxed and comfortable.

People of average weight need about 40 gm of sugar for the insulin effect, those who are heavier may require more.

The following summarises the effect of protein and sugars

food protein →→ ↑ tyrosine and tryptophan in blood →→ albumin in blood binds with tryptophan

→→ proportionally greater levels of tyrosine to tryptophan free in blood

tyrosine is able to enter the brain more freely to form dopamine and noradrenaline, saturating levels and having a stimulating effect

food sugars →→ ↑ blood sugar →→ insulin response causes uptake of blood sugars and amino acids

→→ proportionally greater levels of tryptophan to tyrosine free in blood

tryptophan is able to enter the brain more freely to form serotonin, saturating levels and having a calming effect

Exceptions To The Rule

Saturation

There may be situations where these effects are not as pronounced: this will be when neurotransmitter levels are already saturated in the brain. However modifying your diet will help to maintain the saturated levels and therefore the effect for some time.

Highly Focused Work And Play

When we deplete glucose stores by intense focused activity, we may require carbohydrates to maintain concentration, for example someone who cannot stop playing a video game for hours or someone who has a creative idea they cannot set aside.

A person experiencing a fluctuating intensity of work may require small protein snacks every few hours to maintain dopamine levels and stay alert, providing that the body's glucose stores are not being depleted. A nurse on a night shift of varying intensity is one example.

Restless Nature

In cases where people feel agitated or irritable and find it hard to focus, saturating serotonin through carbohydrates may help them to relax and focus. If they are having difficulty sleeping, ingesting carbohydrates may help prepare them for sleep.

We are all different and some of us naturally more restless than others. Such people may often find that something sweet helps to maintain functioning. They may also be more sensitive to stimulants like coffee, finding that it doesn't take much for their restless nature to come to the surface.

Natural Cycles

We all have natural circadian rhythms, our metabolism tending to be quite slow at dawn and then speeding up quickly over the next few hours. At this time, this natural acceleration means that we will become more attentive anyway and the effect of food may be more limited. This natural rhythm also means a shift towards slowing down from about 4pm, so a carbohydrate meal is likely to have a greater impact towards the evening.

Fat Content

Fat content will increase the length of time required to digest food and will slow you down mentally, because it demands an increased blood flow to the digestive system.

Considerations

Try to minimise fat content when utilising food to control energy levels, especially if wanting to stay alert. A low saturated fat diet is generally a healthy option.

In the case of carbohydrates, don't forget that constantly ingesting sugary foods can cause other health problems, such as fatigue and diabetes. We do not need a lot of sugar for it to have an effect on our mood, so be sensible and try to use starches rather than refined sugars unless you need a very quick effect.

Try to maintain adequate levels of sleep, rest and nutrition. One should ensure adequate intake of vitamins and minerals without relying on food supplements. Vitamins and minerals are required for good mental and physical functioning and are best acquired by eating a varied and healthy diet. This should include fruit, vegetables and nuts, if possible, as well as basic proteins and carbohydrates.

Tyrosine conversion to noradrenaline requires adequate vitamin B12 and zinc (the latter usually deficient in frozen foods). For its conversion to dopamine, it requires vitamins B3 and C, copper and sufficient gastric acid (the acid in one's stomach). Poor digestion, antibiotics and excessive stress can cause some conversion to tyramine, a chemical that can cause anxiety, palpitations, exhaustion and headaches. A healthy balanced diet and a balanced lifestyle should always be a priority.

Useful Information

Most fruits will be high in fructose and are converted slowly to glucose by the body; therefore they do not have the same effect on insulin as foods predominantly composed of glucose. Grapes may be the exception as they are high in glucose.

Foods resulting in a fast insulin response include table sugar and most sweets, as well as honey. The latter should not be cooked but rather added to foods at the end, as it can become toxic (a complementary viewpoint).

Milk, especially skimmed, may behave more like a protein than carbohydrate in its effect.

Remember unless in liquid form, food will take up to a few hours to have an effect, as the body will have to break down solids. The effect may also be delayed if a high fibre meal has been taken.

Fat content will determine to what extent our metabolism slows down and high fat foods should be avoided by most. So be wary of mayonnaise, fried foods, cream and coconut milk in meals.

Exercising enough to raise the heart rate and warm up the body will have a stimulating effect and can keep us alert.

Caffeine

Studies have found that caffeine can improve performance in tasks requiring concentration, complexity and speed reaction(1). Caffeine increases the level of cyclic adenosine monophosphate (cAMP), which is an activator of many neurotransmitters. It does this by inhibiting the chemical phosphodiesterase, which destroys cAMP. The overall effect is to increase levels of many neurotransmitters and alertness.

A reasonably strong cup of coffee, approx 50mg of caffeine and upwards, in the morning can be enough to improve concentration levels for up to four hours or more; further cups in that time will not have a major impact on concentration but can cause physical restlessness and anxiety by their effect on the sympathetic nervous system. For this reason, coffee should be utilised with due consideration as regular use may not suit everyone.

We tend to be more susceptible to the stimulating effect of caffeine after a period of abstinence, such as sleep. In most cases having another cup around 4pm may help us stay alert as our circadian rhythm begins to slow us down. If we are working hard, accompanying this with a few biscuits or something similar may help us to stay alert, by providing the brain with glucose. If you really want to be efficient, remember to take a break, meditate or practise cardiac coherence and then think about caffeine.

Other caffeine containing substances are tea and cocoa, with the latter likely to contain smaller amounts of caffeine. Soft drinks like cola can have as much caffeine as a cup of coffee, but remember to consider the effect of sugar in standard cola drinks.

High doses of caffeine can result in the release of glucose from stores in the liver, resulting in insulin release, which may mean cycles of highs and lows.

Once you monitor the effects of recommended amounts of protein or carbohydrates at different times, as well as the stimulating effect of caffeine, you should be able to utilise them to suit your needs.

If you are using large amounts of caffeine to ward off chronic fatigue, you will not really be doing yourself any favours. A good look at your lifestyle and nutritional intake as well as rest and relaxation strategies may be required.

Using caffeine in this way may well add to your fatigue and stress in the long term. In some cases it may also cause mood swings. In excess, it can drop plasma levels of tyrosine. Very high doses of caffeine can result in an increase in the stress hormone cortisol(2).

There is no substitute for a balanced lifestyle to achieve good health and function. Remember the ultradian rhythms and the need for regular breaks and promotion of cardiac coherence.

Chocolate

Chocolate contains caffeine, tyrosine and phenylalanine. The latter is another precursor to noradrenaline. Chocolate as well as acting as a stimulant, can help restore endorphins, the body's natural painkillers and helps suppress the increase in serotonin after carbohydrate meals, by a decreased glucose and insulin response(3). Dark chocolate high in cocoa and low in sugar will be best for this effect.

Jet Lag

The above concepts may be used to help minimise the effects of travelling through time zones, by influencing the mind and body to stay awake or slow down, in order to synchronise with the time zone at your destination.

Your preparation could start with the meal before your flight by utilising the dopamine or serotonin effect and also making use of caffeine. The aim should be to synchronise your state with the time zone you are heading to, by the time you arrive there. Remember exercise can initially make you feel more alert and awake.

You may want to start resetting your body clock a few days before. This could be done by waking up a few hours earlier or later, depending on the time zone of your destination. Utilising a dawn simulation alarm clock may help (see the section winter blues).

What's On The Menu?

Protein sources of tyrosine that will help with a dopamine and noradrenaline response should be low in fat, such as:
- Egg whites (better) or whole eggs, avoid fried.

- Sea and freshwater fish, including shellfish.

- Skinless chicken and turkey.

- Beef, lamb, mutton or goat, if lean and fat trimmed.

- Veal and venison.

- Lentils, beans and peas.

- Soya and tofu.

- Low fat cottage cheese. Hard cheeses are higher in fats and will not be as effective. Better choices are mozzarella, ricotta and feta.

- Low fat yoghurt and skimmed milk.

Other foods that contain tyrosine - these may not have the same effect on mood as protein sources, but will help in making sure there are adequate supplies in the body. This may be useful in stress related depression. These include:

- Apricot, apple, banana, cherries, fig, strawberries and watermelon.

- Asparagus, avocado, beetroot, carrot, cucumber, lettuce, parsley, red and green peppers, spinach and watercress.

- Almond and peanut.

- Baked beans.

Remember that you can have a little carbohydrate after you have had some protein and still get the dopamine effect. This should probably not be more than the equivalent of a handful of rice. Sashimi and sushi would be appropriate protein choices, as might low fat meat or seafood dishes, followed by some salad and a small amount of complex carbohydrate, e.g. rice or boiled potatoes.

Large meals may slow you down, taking longer to digest, so use moderation when wanting to stay alert.

Fatty meats like pork, most hard cheeses, full fat yoghurt and milk, as well as animal organs, are generally not good sources of low fat protein.

Carbohydrates may be simple or complex, the latter including starches that the body breaks down into simple sugars, including glucose. Starches are generally healthier for the body but will take longer to digest and have an effect on insulin release.

Simple sugars include:

- Sweets and biscuits.
- Jellies and jams.
- Ice creams, try to choose low fat options.
- Soft drinks, beware the caffeine content in some.
- Starches include: rice, pasta, corn, bread and potatoes (avoid fried forms).

Remember that there needs to be enough tryptophan in the body to have the serotonin effect after insulin release. The following foods contain tryptophan. Eating them will not necessarily cause the serotonin effect by itself, but will ensure adequate supplies of tryptophan in the body.

- Chicken, turkey, beef, fish and egg.
- Beets, broccoli, Brussels sprout, carrot, cauliflower celery, spinach, sweet potato, turnip and watercress.
- Cottage, cheddar, parmesan cheeses and milk.
- Oats, pumpkin, sesame and sunflower seeds.
- Banana, date and mango.
- Food is our source of nourishment and should also be a major source of enjoyment. We should try and use meal times as opportunities to practice mindfulness and savour the whole process. Thinking of food as a way to affect our brain chemistry should not change that. In the next section there are further dietary considerations from a complementary perspective.

Key Points

- When eaten alone or at the start of a meal, low fat protein foods can help to keep you alert.

- Carbohydrate foods can help to make you feel calmer and prepare you for sleep. They will have a stronger impact in the evening.

- If you are agitated, carbohydrates may help you focus.

- Use complex carbohydrates if possible. If you want a quick effect, liquid sources will be more suitable. Liquid proteins will also act faster.

- Use caffeine containing foods and drinks sparingly.

- Always think about low fat healthy balanced options.

- Take adequate rest.

Living In The Triangle

We live in a time in which technology allows us to create stable environments, through the use of heating, air conditioning and thermostats. We have car wipers that react to rain drops and shutters that can react to light. Our body and mind are also amazing in their ability to maintain stability, craving certain foods to replenish sugars and proteins and giving out signals so we can put on warm clothing when it is cold or take off a layer when warm.

Our increased understanding of our environment and self allows us to make decisions that facilitate a stable internal and external environment. At the same time we are all different. Some of us feel warmer than others in the same space; some are more sensitive to light or sounds. The same applies to our preferences for food or activities. Some appear more patient, others easily irritated, some more restless, others calm. Some show more determination and drive whilst others seem not to care too much about targets or achievement.

Wouldn't it be great if we could have a working model to explain some of our individual tendencies? Here I want to explore a model that may be of use in giving us a framework for some of our differences and hopefully allow us to engage therapeutically with our environment, helping to facilitate a sense of balance as well as promote a better understanding of one another.

I am referring to the complementary model of Ayurveda: meaning life-knowledge, it originates from the Indian sub-continent and is the oldest of the complementary health systems.

Ayurveda has developed over time and is now taught in the east along with conventional anatomy, physiology and pharmacology. It has influenced a number of holistic medical practices, Chinese and Tibetan, to name but two. It incorporates the use of yoga, acupressure, meditation, food, herbs, colours, music and pretty much anything as required.

Ayurveda starts from the premise that we are all different and that life, as well as our sense of reality, is a subjective experience. It also states that given the right time, place and person, anything can be used therapeutically. As such I make no distinction between it and conventional forms of treatment, all of which, given the right circumstances have a role in keeping us whole.

Most acute health problems, such as myocardial infarcts, asthma attacks, epileptic fits or psychosis are well served by modern medicine, as are many surgical needs, which Ayurveda at one time contributed to greatly, progressing as far as developing caesarean section birth techniques.

The use of Ayurveda as a different way to look at our interaction with the world around us is not based on any judgement of other complementary practices; it is simply the one I am most qualified to speak about here. Those familiar with other complementary practices will in all likelihood be able to appreciate common themes shared by the different systems.

Given the conventional exploration of the subject matter discussed so far, the reader may be surprised at the inclusion of this complementary system. Where Ayurveda can be of use is in helping us engage with our environment on an individual level, providing a potentially versatile approach to help maintain balance. This can be particularly useful in helping us appreciate how, for example, the same food may have a different impact on two different people.

There are numerous texts on the subject and here I propose only to set out an introduction, with an emphasis on our individual predispositions, daily and seasonal cycles, as well as Ayurveda's unique approach regarding the effects of taste and food classification.

Complex problems will best be served by consultation with an appropriate practitioner and those wanting to explore Ayurveda in depth should consult detailed books on the subject.

If some of the following appears esoteric, I would suggest viewing it, in the words of Einstein, as "a model and not a god given truth". All models are subject to reinterpretation and it becomes interesting when this leads to a better understanding of a phenomenon.

An example would be the use of sweet foods in Ayurveda to reduce agitation, which we have already discussed from a conventional neurochemical perspective. Another would be the concept in Ayurveda that suggests stresses are first "processed" by the heart and then the mind, which directs us back to the idea of cardiac coherence aiding neocortical processing, through Ayurvedic practices such as meditation.

If we are ever able to measure all the differences between us, including our different responses to the same situation, we may be surprised how much "different" models may actually have in common once reinterpreted. Most of all, a good model should be effective in its use, and this you will decide for yourself as you apply it.

For people being introduced to Ayurveda for the first time, the following information may seem a lot to take on board. It requires a degree of familiarity and patience to make good use of its concepts. A helpful approach may be to try and understand the underlying principles and use listings such as foods for reference.

What's Your Constitution?

Below we will explore our individual constitution through a questionnaire to see what our inherent "tridoshic" state might be. To ascertain this, answers should reflect our inherent traits, even though we may have moderated them by our diet or activities. Note your total out of each column to get the ratio. If you keep finding yourself regularly undecided between two columns, alternate between the two.

Questions	Answers		
Is your weight	low, little fat	average	heavy
Is your frame	thin	medium	thick
Are your teeth	sharp, irregular	moderate	big, regular
Are your eyes	small, dark	moderate, piercing	large with thick lashes
Is your skin	cool, dry, rough, dark	smooth, soft, light freckled	cool, thick, oily
Is your hair	light & brittle, split ends, curly	moderate, greying early	thick, oily, wavy
Is your forehead	narrow	medium	broad
Is your nose	narrow	medium	broad
Are your lips	narrow, dark	medium, red	broad, pink
Are your actions	active, restless	moderate, precise	slow, methodical
Is your appetite	erratic	strong, irritable when not eating on time	slow & steady
Is your thirst	variable	heavy	light

Are your stools	dry, constipated	soft, regular	heavy, oily
Is your mental disposition	restless, anxious excitable	determined, aggressive, irritable	thoughtful, calm, relaxed
Observation and memory	observant but forgetful	sharp, clear memory	less observant, good memory
Is your speech	talkative & inconsistent	moderate & precise	slow & thoughtful
Is your sleep	poor & erratic	regular	prolonged & sound
Sensitivity to types of weather	cold & dry	heat	cold & damp
Do you spend	impulsively	sensibly	prefer saving
Immunity	poor	moderate	good

The three columns reflect inherent characteristics that make up our constitution. Each column reflects certain clusters that together form vata, pitta and kapha respectively. These are the three "doshas".

Everybody has a different tridoshic state, depending on the ratio of the three doshas. People scoring predominantly from the first column would be vata types, or if scoring equally from the first and second column, vata / pitta. Depending on your constitution, you will be more susceptible to certain illnesses or emotions. Everybody has some degree of all three doshas, as all are required for proper functioning.

Ayurveda views the world as being composed of five elements or types of energy that come together as building blocks to form all things. The differing composition of these elements in all things influences form and function. They are described in a much

43

abbreviated manner here.

"Ether / Space"
This can be regarded as space, between planets or atoms, the canvas on which life occurs. It is regarded as having a nuclear energy.

"Air"
Governs all movement both inside and outside of us. It has an electrical energy, e.g. nerve impulses leading to movement of muscles. Even the revolving of planets is governed by this energy.

"Fire"
Movement and friction lead to fire, which governs all transformation e.g. the digestion of food, the assimilation of knowledge and the registering of information by our senses. It has a radiant, thermal energy.

"Water"
Governs all biochemical functions, acts as a solvent for many substances and has a chemical energy.

"Earth"
All solid, dense materials are derived from this, rocks, muscle and fat. It has a mechanical energy.

These elements are both inside and outside of us. They are normally in a state of harmony, but when significantly disturbed can affect life negatively, whether the death of a planet or the growth of a tumour.

In Ayurveda the five elements are further combined to give form the three doshas. The doshas in turn may be used to describe people, activities, times of day and seasons. They are also associated with colours and can act as a classification system for food. Most animate and inanimate things could be viewed as a ratio of vata, pitta and kapha.

Qualities Of The Doshas

Vata

Composed of ether and air, vata is responsible for all movement, from nerve impulses to movement of food in the gastrointestinal tract. The primary site of residence in the body is the large intestine, others being bone, ear and skin. It has the following attributes: cold, dry, mobile, penetrating, rough, brittle and clear.

Vata types of people may be slim, have sharp or somewhat irregular features with bony prominences and may have a fast metabolism. They may be quick to grasp new concepts but be somewhat forgetful. They may be prone to anxiety or fear. Appetites may be erratic and they should eat when hungry. They may be prone to bloating or flatulence if eating when not hungry and may suffer from constipation due to the drying effect of vata.

Menstruation may be light and irregular.

Vata will be exacerbated by a cold, dry climate or time of year (autumn) as well as cold, dry and raw foods, especially those that are bitter or astringent in taste. Most stimulants such as coffee, tea, ecstacy, amphetamines and cocaine will exacerbate vata.

Vata activities are: fast paced sports e.g. running, flying, driving and excessive exercise or nocturnal activities without suitable rest and nourishment.

Vata time of the day peaks around 4am and 4pm.

Vata time of life is old age, when wasting and dryness become more prominent.

Vata colours are predominantly brown and black and exposure to them may increase vata.

Symptoms of extreme vata imbalance are: feeling cold, pain (unless inflammatory), dryness of skin, palpitations, agitation, anxiety, fear, tiredness and fatigue.

Moisturising, hot baths, sweating, avoiding bitter and astringent foods and using more sweet, salty and sour foods can help to address these symptoms. Calm relaxing activities and rest will also pacify vata agitation.

Pitta

Composed of fire and water, Pitta is responsible for all metabolic processes, from digestion of food to the "digestion" of information by the senses. It has the qualities of being smooth, oily, hot, penetrating, liquid, light or heavy depending on the ratio of fire to water. It is responsible for the lustre of skin, to a "killing look". The primary site is the upper part of the gastrointestinal tract and then blood, eyes, skin and the intellect (head).

Pitta types of people will usually be fair, well proportioned, with symmetrical features. They may be conscious of their appearance and well dressed. They may be methodical, almost obsessive in their style, intelligent and competitive. Emotionally they are prone to anger and irritation.

They are likely to have a strong and fast digestive system, needing to eat when hungry, otherwise becoming irritable. They are more likely to suffer from disorders of the upper gastrointestinal tract e.g. indigestion. Stools are usually soft and regular.

Menstruation is usually regular and may involve heavy periods.

Pitta will be exacerbated by hot climates, summer time, and spicy and sour foods. Many fruits tend to be acidic and will exacerbate pitta. The exceptions are fruits that are very sweet. Most spirits and wines are pitta.

Pitta activities involve exposure to excessive heat, artificial light or working in competitive or goal driven environments.

Pitta times of day peak around 12 noon and midnight. Eating close to midday will help digestion so the main meal should be taken around this time. Cold, heavy foods will be harder to digest as the sun goes down or in the winter, when hot food is more appropriate. The heat of the sun is regarded as making it easier to digest food, by increasing pitta.

Pitta time of life is through our working life from about age 16 to the end of the sixth decade. In these years we may exhibit pitta qualities more strongly e.g. competitiveness, especially if our inherent constitution is pitta.

Pitta colours are predominantly red, then orange, yellow and to a lesser extent green. Exposure to them may increase pitta.

Symptoms of pitta imbalance are inflammatory conditions such as indigestion, tension headaches, excessive sense of heat, sweating, feeling thirsty, excessive appetite, irritation and anger.

Moisturising, cold and sweet foods, eating regularly and exposure to calm water such as lakes and ponds can help to address these. Removing oneself from an over competitive, target driven environment will also help to alleviate pitta problems.

Kapha

Composed of water and earth, Kapha is responsible for giving bulk and support to the body. It is predominant in muscle and fat, helps lubricate joints, aids immunity and supports mental calmness. Its qualities are oily, cold, heavy, slow, dense, slimy, soft and smooth.

Its primary site is the lungs and it is also found in the stomach, joints, heart and brain.

Kapha types tend to be well-built, muscular and often have thick hair and large eyes. They may move slowly, taking their time and are usually accomplished at sports, having good endurance. They may be emotionally prone to attachment and depression. If inactive they are likely to put on weight more easily than vata or pitta types.

Their digestion may be slow, they may need less to eat and they are more prone to disorders of the respiratory system, associated with excessive mucus and congestion e.g. coughs, colds and lung disorders. Stools may be less frequent, heavy and oily.

Menstruation is usually moderate and regular.

Kapha will be exacerbated by a cold, damp climate and the winter season. Also by sweet and salty foods as well as de
nse foods such as dairy, red meats and very dense seafood. Beer will increase phlegm and kapha.

Kapha time of day peaks around 8am and 8pm, when our metabolism is slower.

Kapha time of life is from birth to age 16.

Kapha colours are predominantly light, white and then blue, these being quite calming.

Kapha activities are a sedentary lifestyle, excessive eating and sleeping.

Symptoms of excessive kapha imbalance are sluggishness, lack of motivation, over attachment, excessive weight gain, depression and a propensity to respiratory disorders.

Increased activity, strenuous exercise, sweating, avoiding cold, as well as, sweet, salty and very dense foods will help to address these. Using spicy, sour foods and spirits or wine in moderation will help to alleviate kapha.

Navigating The Triangle

These profiles are a way to look at the interaction of our natural predispositions, present at birth but influenced by our time of life, the time of day, seasons, climate, diet and activities. All of these are in a state of flux and by being aware of the different influences we can try and stay close to a balanced state. Ironically Buddha is reported to have said that he was in a total state of balance for the sum total of three days over his lifetime, so don't be surprised if a little readjustment is the norm!

Most of us will have an inherent ratio of all three doshas. For most people there may be two doshas more strongly expressed, for some only one and rarely all three in equal ratios that is bi, mono or tridoshic.

For example, if we are pitta / kapha in equal proportions, we may have to look out for an excess of pitta in the summer and an excess of kapha in the winter, when these doshas are prominent in our environment. At such times we will have to learn to change our diet and lifestyle to compensate for this, as it is not possible to eat and do the same things all year round, without causing imbalance. Tridoshic people tend to be rare and relatively stable, as their constitution allows them to adapt to changes more easily. If however they shift out of balance, they can be harder to treat.

To understand this better, think of the three doshas as a triangle, with each corner representing purely vata, pitta and kapha respectively. Depending on your constitution, you can pick a point within the triangle to represent your tridoshic state. Time, season, environment, activities and foods consumed, as well as pretty much everything else, will be pulling you towards one of the corners of the triangle.

These forces are in a constant state of flux. By understanding what forces are dominant at any given time and how they interact, we can influence our position in the triangle through food, activities, use of light, music or anything else we like, enabling us to move towards any corner we choose.

Whilst we are born with certain tendencies and a tridoshic state, our decisions and lifestyle will influence how this ratio presents on a day-to-day level. Hence the vata person can become more pitta or kapha and so on.

This concept can be summarised below.

Ether & air.
Cold, dry, penetrating, rough, brittle, clear.
Fast metabolism, bloating, flatulence, constipation.
Irregular & light menstruation.
Cold, dry, windy climates.
Peaks 4am & 4pm. Old age.
Bitter & astringent foods.
Anxiety, fear, palpitations, tiredness, fatigue, pain.
Stimulants, fast paced activities, inadequate rest, nocturnal activities.
Colours: brown & black.

Vata

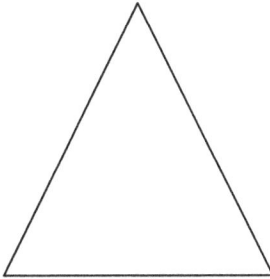

Pitta

Kapha

Fire & water.
Smooth, oily, penetrating, liquid, hot, light or heavy.
Good appetite & metabolism, soft, regular stools dense, soft.
Methodical, obsessive, competitive activities, targets.
Hot climates, summer.
Peaks noon & midnight. 16 to 60.
Regular & heavy menstruation.
Spicy & sour foods, most fruits, spirits & wines.
Anger & irritation. Inflammation.
Colours: red, orange, yellow & green.

Water & earth.
Oily, slimy cold, heavy, slow, dense, soft, smooth.
Well built, slow & steady.
Stools less frequent, oily.
Cold, damp climates, winter.
Regular & moderate menstruation.
Peaks 8am & 8pm.
Birth to 16.
Sedentary lifestyle.
Excessive sleep.
Depression & attachment.
Sweet salty & oily foods.
Colours: white & blue.

Most of us have learnt to select foods and activities that suit us and help facilitate a balanced state. A pitta person may avoid too much spicy and sour food, as well as excessive sunbathing. A kapha person may avoid excessive dense, salty or sweet foods, as well as large meals and will try to stay active. A vata person may try to avoid excessive stimulants and cold and dried foods as well as trying to undertake more calming pastimes.

You will have noticed the interplay of balancing one of the dosha by using the foods and activities from another. The increased kapha in winter could be balanced out by using spicy and pungent foods like chilli, black pepper and ginger, using light therapy or taking a break in a warm climate.

In this way we can also think about treating different conditions. When developing a cold or congestion, which is a kapha condition, we can move away from kapha through increased use of pitta and vata herbs, like lemon, ginger and coriander. When suffering from indigestion or inflammatory conditions, we can decrease pitta and increase kapha or vata by using milk to reduce symptoms of indigestion, or in the case of a swollen painful joint, apply ice to reduce the inflammation.

Derangements of physical and emotional states are not likely to appear unless we lose this mechanism of rebalancing. Sometimes a loss of balance leads to activities that magnify the initial imbalance: for instance, a vata person staying up late into the night, doing things quickly, finding it difficult to slow down and then taking more stimulants and staying up even later, or a kapha person comfort eating sugary foods when already lethargic and inactive.

Another example would be a pitta person becoming very driven and competitive, looking for even more challenges. Note that the "air" of vata may "fan the fire" of pitta. Kapha activities and foods are more likely to help slow down and cool things in pitta types. An example of "fanning the fire" could be rushing around to get things done, as well as being competitive or target driven. The heat of pitta may exacerbate vata by its drying effect.

The Six Tastes

Ayurveda also has a classification system for food based on vata, pitta and kapha. Generally speaking these correspond to taste. Six tastes are recognised and each corresponds to two elements, two tastes belonging to one dosha. This is a unique way to think about the possible effects of foods we are not familiar with.

Vata   Bitter (ether / air) & Astringent (air / earth) like cardamom, clove and tea.

Pitta   Sour (fire / earth) & Pungent (fire / air) like chilli, black pepper or wasabi.

Kapha   Salty (fire / water) & Sweet (water / earth)

Effects Of The Six Tastes

Sweet
Promotes growth of tissues, is soothing to the mind, gives strength and a good complexion, relieves thirst and burning sensations. Excess leads to lethargy, heaviness, obesity, cough, breathing difficulties, weak digestion and increased mucus.

Sour
Improves the taste of food, aids swallowing and digestion, awakens the mind, reduces flatus, promotes salivation. Excess may make the teeth sensitive, cause thirst and increase inflammatory conditions.

Salty

Promotes digestion, can work as a sedative and laxative, promotes salivation and adds taste to food. Excess can dull the senses, wrinkle the skin, induce hyperacidity, decrease virility and increase inflammatory conditions.

Pungent

Promotes digestion, purifies food, promotes nasal secretions, causes tears and sharpens the senses. It helps to relieve blood stagnation. Excess causes decreased virility, emaciation, burning and thirst.

Bitter

Restores the sense of taste, detoxifies, can act as an antibacterial and antipyretic. Helps thirst and inflammation, removes toxic accumulations. Excess causes tissue wasting, emaciation, weariness and dryness.

Astringent

Is sedating, stops diarrhoea, helps close and heal sores and wounds. Dries and firms tissues and helps to stop bleeding. Excess causes drying out, constipation, dark skin, decreased virility, premature ageing, flatus, emaciation, thirst and stiffness.

As a general rule people should avoid too much of the food corresponding to their dosha, especially if it is intensified by the time of year, or their activities.

Vata types should avoid excess bitter, astringent and pungent tastes, due to their drying effect, especially in autumn, when vata is predominant. Sweet, sour and salty tastes will be more suitable.

Pitta types should, avoid excess sour, pungent and to a lesser degree salty tastes, as they contain the fire element, especially in the summer. Sweet, bitter and astringent tastes will be more suitable.

Kapha types should avoid excess salty, sweet and to a lesser degree sour tastes, especially in winter, and use bitter, astringent and pungent tastes.

We have already mentioned that most people are likely to be a combination of two predominant doshas and therefore may have to pay more attention to what they avoid. This will depend on which dosha is intensified by the season or climate they find themselves in, as well as upon their activities. The above are general rules and the context of your situation is important.

We all need a little of all tastes in our diet, so it would not be wise to totally eliminate the tastes corresponding to our dosha, but we need to be aware of excess.

Ayurveda considers that the action of foods starts with taste (rasa), of which there are six, as mentioned. It then breaks these down to an initial heating or cooling effect on the body (virya) and then a post digestive effect (vipaka). These are outlined below.

Taste (Rasa)	Hot / Cold (Virya)	Post (Vipaka)
Bitter	Cold	Pungent
Astringent	Cold	Pungent
Pungent	Hot	Pungent
Sour	Hot	Sour
Salty	Hot	Sweet
Sweet	Cold	Sweet

The hot and cold initial effect can be regarded as a thermal response on the body, with the post digestive being a metabolic effect whereby pungent speeds up metabolism and is potentially catabolic (decreasing), sour may be regarded as neutral, and sweet is anabolic (increasing). So, if we do not wish to put on weight easily, we could avoid an excess of salty and sweet tastes in our choice of foods.

As with most things in life, there are exceptions to the rule. In Ayurveda, foods having unorthodox characteristics are termed "Prabhavya".

A few such foods include: turmeric, which is bitter but hot, onions being pungent but cold, lime being sour but cold, whilst a lemon is sour and hot. The latter might explain why a lime usually tastes more refreshing in drinks, especially in the summer.

Suitability of foods for vata, pitta and kapha types are given in the following charts. These are in keeping with the recommendations already made with regards to taste. Recommended foods for a particular dosha will help to reduce that dosha and vice versa.

Use the charts as a reference to ascertain the effects of different foods on the different doshas. These can then be used to increase or decrease vata, pitta or kapha.

	Vata	Pitta	Kapha
Meats	Most meats are good for vata, especially fish, beef, most shellfish, the darker meat of chicken & turkey. Avoid pork, lamb, mutton & drier meats like rabbit & venison.	White meats and freshwater fish are good, as is venison. Most red meats will exacerbate pitta as will the larger seafood and most shellfish. Shrimps are acceptable in moderation.	Dark white meats, seafood and red meat will exacerbate kapha. White chicken, turkey, freshwater fish, shrimp, venison & rabbit are acceptable.
Eggs	Good	Avoid yolks; egg white is acceptable.	Acceptable if not fried.
Dairy	Generally good, but take care with powdered milks & very cold products like ice cream. Hard cheeses in moderation.	Salted and sour dairy products will exacerbate pitta, including fruit yoghurts & hard cheeses. Soft young cheeses, ice cream & fresh yoghurt with water are acceptable in moderation.	Generally avoid. Salted dairy, butter, ice cream, most cheeses & yoghurt will exacerbate kapha. Skimmed milks, occasional cottage cheese & diluted yoghurt may be acceptable.
Grains	Rice, wheat and oats preferably cooked. Rice cakes in moderation. Avoid bran, barley, granola, millet & dried oats.	Yeast containing grain foods like bread can increase pitta, along with corn, millet & dry oats. Bran, rice, barley and granola are better choices.	Dry oats, corn, barley, bran, millet are acceptable, i.e. the drier grains.
Nuts raw and lightly roasted are heavy, nourishing and hard to digest.	Small amounts of peeled almond, walnut, pecan & pine soaked overnight are acceptable.	Coconut, sunflower as well as small amounts of almond & sesame, soaked overnight are acceptable.	Sunflower & pumpkin are acceptable.

57

	Vata	Pitta	Kapha
Legumes	Red and green lentils are good also soy cheese, soymilk, soy sauce & tofu. Avoid soybeans, dried peas, kidney, black beans & black lentils.	Miso and soy is pitta exacerbating. Other legumes are acceptable.	Most lentils, chickpeas, black beans, soymilk, dried peas & heated tofu are acceptable. Avoid other forms of soy, cold tofu, kidney & butter beans.
Vegetables	Avoid dried and frozen foods. Broccoli, peppers cauliflower, eggplant, winter squashes, mushrooms & celery will exacerbate vata. Most cooked vegetables are good. Summer squashes, sweet potato, parsnip, pumpkin, onions (cooked), asparagus, green beans & occasionally spinach are acceptable, as are sweet & watery vegetables e.g. cucumber.	Avoid pungent & acidic vegetables, like tomatoes, raw onions, red peppers & raw beets. Cooked spinach with e.g. olive oil occasionally is acceptable. Most bitter & sweet vegetables will help reduce pitta e.g. cucumbers, leafy greens, mushrooms, green peppers, carrots, cooked beets, broccoli, celery, cabbage, cauliflower, asparagus, potatoes, squashes, sprouts & cooked onion.	Generally better to take warm & with spices. Sweet and watery vegetables will exacerbate kapha. So cucumber, zucchini, sweet potatoes & tomatoes should be avoided. Bitter & pungent vegetables are good for kapha types e.g. peppers, leafy greens, sprouts, broccoli, asparagus, peas, cabbage, eggplant & celery.
Oils	Apart from flax seed, most oils will alleviate vata. Sesame, ghee, olive oil, sunflower & canola oil are acceptable for cooking. Coconut oil is a heavy oil & good for external use.	Almond, sesame and corn oil are heating in nature and will aggravate pitta. Ghee, canola, olive & sunflower oil are good for cooking & coconut externally.	Avoid most oils except the lighter, heating ones. Corn, sunflower & canola are good for cooking, with sesame being good externally due to its rough quality.

	Vata	Pitta	Kapha
Fruit	Most dried forms of fruits will exacerbate vata. Soaked prunes or raisins are acceptable as are most sweet fruit & some sour fruits e.g. grapes, sweet melons, bananas, oranges, grapefruit, lime, lemon, mangoes, peaches, plums & pineapple.	Sour fruit is acidic, it can exacerbate pitta. These fruits can include plums, berries, apples, cherries, peaches, pineapple, oranges & bananas. Sweet, pineapple, oranges, berries & plums are acceptable. Figs, sweet melon, lime, raisins, prune & pears are acceptable. Lemons & green grapes may also aggravate pitta.	Sweet, sour, denser & very watery fruits are best avoided e.g. dates, bananas, mangoes, melon, pineapple, & plums. Lighter & drier fruit are good e.g. prunes raisins, pears, apples peaches, cherries. Some watery acidic fruits like limes, lemons, strawberries & grapes are acceptable in moderation.
Spices	Most spices will be good: however be careful of the drying effect of chilli & black pepper if used excessively.	Cayenne, cloves, garlic, nutmeg, oregano, dry ginger, mustard seeds & asafoetida are all heating & best avoided. Coriander, cumin, turmeric, cinnamon, saffron, fennel, parsley, fresh ginger & a little black pepper are acceptable.	Apart from salt, all spices are good for kapha types.
Sweeteners White sugar is to be generally avoided.	Apart from white sugar, most are acceptable e.g. honey, molasses, rice syrup & maple syrup in moderation.	Avoid molasses. Honey in moderation due to its heating effect. Most others are acceptable.	Honey & fruit juice concentrates are acceptable, avoid others.

	Vata	Pitta	Kapha
Beverages Iced drinks are generally not recommended. They may cause vasoconstriction resulting in difficulty digesting. If taken, they are best consumed in warmer climates and not with meals.	Stimulating, drying fizzy & very cold drinks should be avoided e.g. spirits, red wine, cranberry, apple juice, caffeinated drinks, ginseng & dandelion teas. Be wary of other bitter or astringent teas. Orange pineapple, grape, mango & pineapple juices are acceptable. So are cider, beer & white wine. Fennel, liquorice, rosehip & peppermint are good choices for herbal teas.	Avoid caffeinated & cocoa drinks, spirits & red wine. Most acidic fruit juices will exacerbate pitta & the same rule applies for fruits. This includes most berries. Tomato juice will exacerbate pitta. Pomegranate, grape & prune juices, along with sweet orange, almond, soy & rice milk are acceptable. Herbal teas of camomile, fennel, dandelion, liquorice are good, but ginseng will exacerbate pitta.	Beer, sweet wine, dairy based, highly salted & very sweet drinks are best avoided. Astringent drinks like pomegranate & cranberry are good as are grape & prune juice. So is soymilk if spiced. Stimulating or light teas e.g. black tea, cinnamon, mints & chamomile as well as corresponding fruit teas are good. A little caffeine is acceptable.

Food And Mind In Ayurveda

Ayurveda categorises foods based on their effect on the mind. It uses three categories, Sattva, Rajas and Tamas.

Sattvic foods are regarded as promoting a calm insightful mind, love, forgiveness and compassion.

Rajasic foods may in excess contribute to fear, anger, jealousy and envy. These are often strongly vata or pitta.

Tamasic foods may in excess contribute to attachment, dullness, depression and drowsiness. These may be strongly kapha.

The degree to which you are affected will depend on your mental and physical state as well as your predispositions. A sattvic state could be regarded as "equidistant" between vata, pitta and kapha.

Meats
No meats are regarded as intensifying sattvic qualities. Seafood, especially shellfish and larger fish are rajasic, so is chicken, with other heavier (red) meats being regarded as tamasic in the long term.

Legumes
Red, green and yellow lentils are sattvic. Most beans will be rajasic in small doses and tamasic in large doses. Black lentils are tamasic.

Herbs
Saffron, turmeric, cumin, coriander, fennel and cardamom are sattvic. These herbs are also good for aiding digestion without exacerbating pitta and related conditions such as indigestion. Chillis and black pepper are rajasic with nutmeg and jalapeno

peppers being tamasic.

Grains
Basmati rice and barley are sattvic, with heavier or brown rice being tamasic. Corn and millet are rajasic.

Vegetables
Leafy greens, asparagus, zucchini, sprouts, sweet potatoes and summer squashes are sattvic. Winter squashes, broccoli, potatoes, spinach and most pickled vegetables are rajasic. Mushroom, garlic and pumpkin are tamasic.

Fruits
Generally fruits are regarded as sattvic, especially figs, dates, pomegranates, coconut and pears. Very sour fruits may be somewhat rajasic, with avocado and honeydew melon being tamasic.

Dairy
Organic goat's milk, cow's milk and yoghurt are sattvic. Sour cream, softer cheeses and ice cream are rajasic. Processed milk, hard and aged cheese are tamasic.

Nuts
Almonds, fresh cashews and white sesame seeds are sattvic, with most other nuts being rajasic, except peanuts, which are tamasic.

Sugars
Raw honey and fresh sugarcane juice are sattvic, most processed sugars rajasic and really sweet tasting foods such as processed sweets, chocolates and cakes are tamasic. Dark chocolate with a high cocoa content may be rajasic.

Teas
Liquorice tea is sattvic, coffee, black and green teas are rajasic.

Illicit Drugs
Most illicit stimulants are rajasic, but marijuana is tamasic in the long term.

Alcohol
May be rajasic, but excess use will be tamasic.

A Little Discussion Of The Food Charts

Having gone through the chart, you may be shaking your head, thinking about all the foods you should be avoiding. The charts basically tell you how foods affect the three doshas. If you continually exacerbate your inherent dosha, you may get away with things for a while, but in the long term, you will begin to experience problems related to an excess of that dosha.

If you are going to start changing your eating habits, do so gradually, as your body needs time to adapt from what it is used to.

Providing you use moderation and a balanced approach, you can from time to time eat a food that would normally exacerbate your dosha. A wise course would be to introduce another food or herb that will balance out the effect of that particular food. It may also be worth taking the time of day and the season into consideration.

In the case of a pitta person who likes prawns, the use of spinach cooked with prawns and coconut milk with cooler spices will alleviate some of the heating effect of prawns, especially if eaten in winter.

Occasional consumption of heavier meats or seafood by a kapha person may be acceptable if using strong spices that alleviate kapha. Eating closer to midday might also be advisable.

Another example could be an occasional cup of coffee with cardamom, in the winter by a vata person.

You can usually find a way of balancing your food intake by considering the density, texture, taste and colour of ingredients.

Generally speaking the more you try to keep your inherent dosha in check, the more likely you are to avoid future problems and to feel balanced in mind and body.

For those of us who may want to lose weight and have a predominant kapha dosha, useful measures would be to increase vata and pitta foods and avoid kapha foods. Aim to eat a light breakfast after 10am, as you go from kapha to pitta time of day and your metabolism speeds up. Have your main meal around 1-2pm and if required, a lighter evening meal around 6-7pm, before the next kapha cycle begins.

Using strong pungent and bitter spices in cooking will also help kapha types, as will only sipping a suitable beverage with food. Cold and watery salads lacking bitter or pungent ingredients are best avoided, especially in winter, as they will act as water to dilute gastric juices.

The result of following these suggestions will be to help the digestion, without slowing down the metabolism. Exercise will also help speed up one's metabolism. Pitta types wanting to lose weight should use spices that are less heating to the body, so as not to exacerbate pitta (see the food charts).

Good digestion of food in Ayurveda will depend on its suitability for you and your eating habits. Ayurveda views incomplete digestion of food as leading to toxin formation, which if it continues to accumulate over time will lead to chronic diseases. The concept of complete digestion in Ayurveda means attaining a light satisfied state after a meal, in keeping with optimal functioning.

The right food for you as an individual, at the right time, with you in the right frame of mind to receive it, is regarded as highly important to achieve a healthy balance for both mind and body.

We live in changing environments, so using the Ayurvedic categorisation of food can also be a useful way of enhancing our mental and physical state. Utilise kapha foods to calm yourself or slow down (sugars saturating serotonin), pitta foods when needing to stay focused and vata when needing to feel more active. Bear in mind that excess of kapha, pitta and vata foods will lead to lethargy, irritation or anxiety, respectively, especially if it conforms with your constitution.

Eating appropriately for your constitution and current state will have a number of beneficial effects. It may also be useful to take some other factors into consideration. These are explored in the next section.

Some Rules For Eating & Drinking

Time
Make time to eat. Being distracted by work, loud music, excessive conversation or the television is unlikely to be helpful. Be mindful and savour every mouthful. It takes time for your mind to register that you have had enough to eat, so taking your time should prevent overeating and unnecessary weight gain. Try to avoid getting so hungry that you end up overeating. If this occurs regularly try taking a little snack or fruit between meals, perhaps during an ultradian break.

Place
Try to be sitting in a pleasant environment, with pleasant company if possible. Avoid eating at your desk or when walking.

State
If you find yourself in a charged emotional state, allow yourself time to calm down and eat later. Ingesting a sweet, non-stimulating beverage may help to achieve this. Eating whilst emotionally charged is likely to hinder digestion.

Source
Whenever possible, make sure you know where your food is coming from, who prepared it and with what intention. Food should be made with love and care. If that is not possible, try to buy food from places that aspire to quality.

Freshness
Whenever possible, eat freshly prepared food, with the minimum of additives or preservatives. Try to avoid frozen (these tend to be deficient in zinc) and canned foods if possible.

Microwaves
Try to avoid microwaves for cooking and warming up.

Six Tastes
Make sure your meals have at least a trace of all six tastes, as a deficiency may leave you dissatisfied and still hungry, even if you have had large portions. This is the curse of most fast food.

Water
Only sip water or a recommended beverage with your food, preferably at room temperature. Excessive water will dilute your gastric juices and cold water will cause vasoconstriction resulting in reduced blood flow, further slowing digestion. This will lead to the increased likelihood of toxins being formed as well as a propensity to put on weight.

Proteins
More than two forms of protein at a time may make it harder for the body to digest the food properly. Ideally just have one form and try to avoid heavy protein meals in the evening. They are best taken earlier in the day.

Dairy / Meat
Having dairy products and meat together will make digestion that much slower and harder. If combining these, use a lot of herbs and spices to aid digestion. Ideally eat such combinations earlier in the day.

Dairy / Seafood
Ayurveda considers certain food combinations to be difficult to digest and to increase the risk of toxins forming. These include mixing any seafood with dairy products. Coconut milk is acceptable and may be used instead.

Sweet / Sour
Excessively sweet and sour dishes are also best avoided for similar reasons.

Stages
Ayurveda breaks digestion into six stages, corresponding to tastes. Starting with sweet then sour, pungent, salty, bitter and lastly astringent. Ideally foods corresponding to these tastes should be eaten close to this order where possible. Some cultures do this by starting with bread, crackers or poppadoms and may end the meal with a tea, which has an astringent taste. If you need to work straight after lunch, you may want to make use of the food and mood strategies discussed earlier and start with proteins.

Some schools of thought suggest that a little sweet food is acceptable at the end of your meal. I suggest you use your own judgement and consider the choice of food. For example, instead of having a portion of ice cream, which is cold, likely to cause vasoconstriction and slow down digestion, you may be better off with a little dark chocolate instead. It may satisfy your desire for a sweet taste as well as being bitter. Dark chocolate may also reduce serotonin saturation, helping to keep you alert and restore the body's endorphins.

Tea / Coffee
Avoid stimulating drinks like tea or coffee before meal times, as their stimulating effect is likely to reduce blood flow to the gastrointestinal system. It may be better to consume these a short while after your food, when they are more likely to aid digestion.

Hunger
Only eat when you are ready. Generally, vata types should eat when hungry, pitta types regularly to avoid the build up of acid in an empty stomach and feelings of irritation. Kapha types should try

to avoid eating at kapha times of day. Ideally try to have your main meal around midday, as it will be more easily digested. Most Buddhist monks eat once a day at lunchtime.

Evening Meal
Try to eat evening meals about four hours before you go to bed, as eating later will mean food in your stomach when lying down, making you more prone to acid reflux as well as slowing the digestion. If needed, choose a light snack or drink closer to bedtime. A light carbohydrate snack may help you relax and prepare for sleep. Proteins generally take longer to digest and are best eaten earlier in the day.

Digestion
Once you have eaten a reasonable meal, your metabolism will dictate how long it takes for food to digest. This can take anything up to five hours depending on who, what, when and where. If you haven't digested your last meal, eating another meal in this time will confuse your body, which is at a different stage of digestion and not primed to start another cycle. It will lead to poor digestion and the production of toxins.

If necessary, take appropriate snacks after a few hours; fruits are good, or a few biscuits with tea if you are working hard. Some people, especially pitta types, may benefit from smaller more regular meals. Remember to heed your ultradian rhythms when considering the timing of your food.

Fruit
Fruit with meals can lead to excess acidity and it is usually best taken on its own, as are honeydew melons due to their heavy nature. Most fruits contain predominantly fructose with some exceptions, such as grapes, containing glucose. Most are an ideal source of energy and nutrients between meals, helping to keep you

going. Fructose will impact less on your insulin response.

Sweets
Sweets may be better eaten on their own. Taken around teatime, they may impact less on your insulin response and be more quickly digested than when taken after a large meal. If you are working hard, a little something sweet with a cup of tea may help to keep you going.

Insulin
It is now generally accepted that foods that have a low glycaemic index, that is, foods that do not cause high blood sugar levels and a high insulin response after consumption, can help reduce the risk of diabetes and unnecessary weight gain.

Further Ayurvedic Information

Those wanting to explore Ayurveda in more detail may wish to start by exploring books by Dr Vasant Lad, which are available from bookshops and through the internet. Dr Lad is based at the Ayurvedic Institute, Albuquerqe: www.ayurveda.com

The Ayurvedic Practitioners Association in the UK may be contacted for information and local practitioners: www.apa.uk.com

Breaks

If you were told you couldn't have a holiday all year, chances are you would quit your job. We all need time to recuperate, gain some inspiration or just spend time with loved ones. Addressing these needs usually means we are in better health, as well as more energetic and productive at work. Ideally breaks should be at regular intervals and the next one planned as soon as you get back, ensuring you have something to look forward to.

The same philosophy should apply to lunch and weekend breaks. Lunch breaks should not just be about getting something to eat; they should also get you away from work, so you can "process" your morning, maintain your brain chemistry according to your needs and get to practise some mindfulness, whilst enjoying your meal. A lot achieved in a short space of time.

Eating while trying to work is not really constructive, or good for your physical and mental health. Take the break and come back refreshed whenever possible. A good work ethic should not preclude you from taking regular breaks in order to maintain optimal productivity.

Bear in mind that the ultradian rhythms suggest we have a cycle of between 90-120 minutes, during which 20 minutes are required to process what we have been doing. At this time, we are less productive and likely to become emotional and self-critical. We are also likely to become more fidgety.

The best thing we can do is go and take a 20 minute break at these times or engage in less demanding activity. Continuously pushing yourself through these times will cause increasing stress and be counterproductive in the long term.
For those of us who are self employed, ensuring appropriate breaks

and at least a day off every week can sometimes be difficult. However doing so will potentially have great benefits. So if you want to work effectively, try taking regular breaks - and forget the guilt.

Winter Blues

For people some distance from the equator, long nights can have a strong impact on our energy levels, concentration and mood. In some cases people suffer a depression-like illness known as SAD or seasonal affective disorder. This may occur due to the lack of exposure to sunlight or what is known as full spectrum lighting. Most artificial light sources are unable to provide the full spectrum lighting that we require.

In each 24 hour period we are predisposed to be awoken by the increasing intensity of sunlight, drifting in and out of sleep, gradually becoming more alert. This process helps to maintain normal biorhythms, such as the increase in our melatonin hormone levels at night and a decrease in response to light. Unfortunately natural light has been replaced by the obtrusive sound of an alarm and in winter sudden artificial light. On waking, this can leave us feeling sluggish, as melatonin levels have not had a chance to drop.

The lack of a natural dawn can be addressed by using a dawn simulation alarm clock. These devices gradually provide an increasing intensity of light mimicking the dawn and helping to maintain the natural melatonin cycle. Some of these devices work as light sources that can also be used at other times.

For those suffering from seasonal affective disorder (SAD), a full spectrum light source of adequate brightness may be required to alleviate the condition. Adequate exposure time is required, anything from 15-90 minutes a day depending on the individual.

A range of alarms and light boxes are available as well as full spectrum lighting for the home. Some companies such as Sunrise System offer models which combine a light box with a dawn simulation alarm. Such devices may be ordered from a number of suppliers through the internet.

More information on SAD and light therapy can be found on the MIND website, by searching for seasonal affective disorder: www.mind.org.uk

Exercise

Regular exercise, even as little as 20 minutes, three times a week can be enough to improve one's general health. Exercise can act to speed up metabolism and release endorphins, which give a natural high and reduce stress levels. It can also help to maintain good cardiovascular functioning and prevent a relapse into depressive symptoms. According to department of health guidelines, highly intensive exercise regimes are not necessary for these benefits. "Thirty minutes of moderate activity five times a week is all it takes to improve and maintain good health." (www.dh.gov.uk).

It is generally a good idea to warm up before stretching, as you will be less likely to injure yourself, and to warm down after exercising. Warming up may be achieved by a light jog, cycling, rowing or stepper exercises for about 10-15 minutes, followed by stretching. Warming down can be achieved by decreasing the intensity of activity over 10-15 minutes, allowing the body time to slowly cool down.

Do what you enjoy, but also try to have a balance where you work on strength, stamina and suppleness; combining yoga with gym sessions is one example. Many gyms may feature TV screens and loud music. If your day is already quite frantic and affects you adversely, consider more mindful exercises such as swimming or yoga.

If you participate in high impact sports like jogging or squash, minimise damage to joints by wearing good footwear, replacing these before they are too worn to offer good cushioning and where possible run on soft ground.

If you are starting out after a long break, go slowly and if necessary seek some supervision. Be careful not to overdo it, as your body will need time to adjust. It's better to do a little bit regularly than to keep starting and stopping.

Unless you train at high intensity regularly, you should not require food supplements. Adequate fluids during and after exercise and a generally healthy diet should suffice.

If you run regularly or do exercises that are likely to impact on cartilage, tendons and ligaments, you might want to consider glucosamine supplementation, to ensure adequate supplies for remodelling of these tissues. It may be worth consulting a professional for further advice regarding formulations and doses.

Quite often people say that they will take up exercise, proper lunch breaks or meditating when they have time. It may be better to consider putting things in place that keep you well mentally and physically and then taking care of business, rather than waiting till you have time. You will feel more relaxed and may be surprised at how much more efficiently you can function when operating in this way.

Omega-3 Fatty Acids

These fats are present in oily fishes, grass fed animals (not grain) and some plant sources. However their availability in our food may have declined by as much as 20 times due to changes in farming methods. The use of grains in place of grass for animal feed is causing an increase in omega-6 content in animals. An excess of omega-6 can result in inflammatory reactions(1).

Grass fed animals tend to have higher omega-3 levels. These fatty acids are recognised as having an important anti-inflammatory role. Inflammation is involved in a number of illnesses such as cancer, arthritis, Alzheimer's and cardiovascular disease(2). These fatty acids may also contribute towards good mental health.

Three portions a week of oily fish, or an equivalent oily plant source, are thought to be adequate for our requirements. Further supplementation should not normally be required, unless there is a known deficiency.

The following are good sources:

Walnuts, mackerel, tuna, salmon, trout, sardines, anchovies, spinach, flax seeds and oil, rapeseed oil, spirulina and watercress.

Large oily fish like shark and swordfish, whilst high in omega-3, are likely to be contaminated by high levels of mercury. This will be lower in smaller fish. White fish tend to be less oily and lower in omega-3.

Grass fed meat sources are also good and organic eggs can have up to 20 times as much omega-3 as non-organic(3).

Cooking with certain oils will mean competition with other fatty acids for uptake, as most are high in omega-6. The exceptions are canola oil (1/3rd omega-3) and olive oil which is neutral. These will be suitable choices for cooking when wanting to increase omega-3 intake.

Food Supplements And Herbal Remedies

Available in a wide variety of forms, excessive vitamins can be toxic in high doses and if not utilised by the body are usually excreted and not stored. They may also be quite hard to digest. A healthy diet should not normally require supplementation, unless there is a specific deficiency being treated and then probably under medical supervision.

If you are tired and not functioning properly, take a good look at the different aspects of your life before reaching for a quick fix, as it may just mask the real problem. If you take supplements or herbal remedies without medical supervision, consider breaks, rather than prolonged regular use, which will build up tolerance and may make them less effective. In some cases, such as ginseng, a fortnightly cycle of use and breaks may be beneficial.

There are very many herbal products available, ranging from Bach, homeopathic and Chinese to Ayurvedic remedies, to mention just a few. Many complementary systems use a holistic integrated approach when dealing with symptoms. Off the shelf remedies may not address fundamental problems that require the attention of a practitioner.
Some herbs whilst useful, can have serious side effects. For instance the anticoagulant properties of Ginko Biloba can interact with aspirin and prescribed anticoagulants. In the case of St John's Wort, there may be a reduction in the efficacy of oral contraceptive and epileptic medication. Always check for

interactions if on medication.

Some supplements or herbal remedies may be of known benefit and may even be available through your GP on prescription. St John's Wort for depression springs to mind. In such cases, certain formulations are recommended and considered more efficacious. It may be worthwhile getting advice from your doctor or pharmacist.

Alcohol

Current department of health recommendations are the same for men and women and set at 14 units per week. One unit is half a pint of average strength beer, a small glass of wine or sherry and a measure of spirits. In Scotland the spirit measure can be 1.2 units. A bottle of wine (12%) is the equivalent of nine units.

It can be easy to drink more than the recommended amounts and due caution is required. Unfortunately signs of alcohol complications like liver and heart disease can show up quite late, when damage is already advanced.

Excess alcohol can also cause dietary deficiencies through malabsorption of nutrients, especially B vitamins. Other conditions such as anxiety, depression, fatigue, diabetes, obesity and cancers of the mouth, larynx, oesophagus, breast and liver are also linked to excessive consumption.

Anyone who is concerned about his or her use of alcohol should get professional advice. Investigations to ascertain negative impact can be easily arranged through your GP. For those who would like to monitor and address excessive drinking at an early stage, the website www.downyourdrink.org.uk may be of help. There is further advice at www.drinkaware.co.uk

Drugs

Like alcohol, illicit drugs such as cannabis, ecstasy, MDMA, amphetamines, cocaine and opiates can cause serious complications. Cannabis can act on a number of receptors in the brain, with different effects on different people, depending on the type and quantity taken.

Ecstasy and MDMA primarily work through increasing serotonin levels in the brain, with regular use depleting supplies of tryptophan (the precursor amino acid). Amphetamines and cocaine can cause an increase in levels of dopamine, with subsequent depletion of tyrosine (the precursor amino acid). All these stimulants can cause symptoms such as anxiety, insomnia depression, irritability and mood swings.

Many of these drugs may well cause toxicity of the nervous system and possible damage. Regular use of most recreational drugs will build tolerance, resulting in progressively more being required for the same effect. They are likely to cause disruption of normal sleep.

Stimulants will usually increase body temperature, blood pressure and heart rate as well as divert blood from the gastrointestinal system, making digestion more difficult. These effects can result in malnutrition, accelerated breakdown of the body's muscle tissue, increased strain on the kidneys, and heightened risk of a stroke. Cocaine is well known for causing a spasm of blood vessels and can result in reduced blood supply and damage to a number of different parts of the body, including myocardial infarcts and strokes.

Opiates can, when being withdrawn, cause: insomnia, restlessness, increased heart rate and hypertension as well as a host of gastrointestinal problems.

There is also the risk from needle sharing of contracting hepatitis or HIV. Hepatitis C may be contracted by sharing snorting devices.

In vulnerable individuals, most illicit drugs can bring mental illness to the surface. Anyone with such a predisposition will be susceptible to fluctuations in brain chemistry and potential deterioration of their mental state. Amphetamine use is known to cause schizophrenia-like symptoms even in the less vulnerable.

Know the risks and make an informed decision. If you have concerns speak to a professional, such as your local doctor. The websites www.talktofrank.com (0800 77 66 000) in the UK and www.knowthescore.info (0800 587 5879) in Scotland can also be contacted for advice and referral.

Conflict Resolution

One thing that life usually guarantees is that others will upset us. At such times, being mindful and open to other people's reasons for a viewpoint may be useful.

Try to identify potential areas of conflict through consideration of another person's or one's own:
- sense of **identity**
- perceived invasion of **territory**
- sense of having lost **control**
- sense of having an unmet **need**

Examining these may enable you to highlight the underlying nature of the problems and suggest solutions. Huntington suggested the first three areas, after a study of conflict in primary healthcare in 1981.

For any subsequent discussion make sure you choose the right:

Time: consider the person's ultradian rhythm and when they may be more introspective and receptive to discourse or a peace offering. Make sure you have enough time to discuss the matter fully rather than leaving it half finished.

Place: decide is privacy required to avoid any public loss of face?

Person: deal with someone who can actually help address the problem and consider their tridoshic constitution: vata types may benefit from reassurance, pitta from a non-confrontational approach and kapha a little prompting.

If you feel resentment or contempt, consider using the techniques of cardiac coherence and mindfulness rather than responding emotionally. Some calm reflection and meditation may help us to come up with an appropriate coping strategy, or even to accept that we may also need to take some responsibility.

Talking about one's own feelings rather than criticising the other person is an effective way of communicating. It may be useful to frame things in the positive; for example telling someone that it would be better if they did something, rather than telling them what not to do. This usually means they will then imagine the thing they are being asked to do, rather than the thing to avoid. Such requests could be put as "I feel happier when you...".

Try to be friendly in your approach, as people usually mimic each other's style of interaction: a smile usually receives a smile and vice versa with antagonism.

Sleeping Arrangements

A few simple rules can sometimes help promote restful sleep. Wherever possible try to dedicate your bedroom to sleeping. It may be better to work elsewhere. Try to minimise equipment such as computers, televisions or stereos. Make the room, a calm relaxed environment, with suitable colour and décor. Try to use a good bed, pillows and duvet.

It is generally a good idea to go to bed after you have wound down and are feeling a little sleepy, rather than going when alert or stimulated by fast paced music or movies. If it's late and you need to settle down after such activity, try making use of a light sweet drink or snack: saturating serotonin levels may aid you in getting ready for sleep.

Exercise can also help you relax, due to the body's release of natural painkillers, the endorphins, which have a calming sedative-like effect. Remember exercise may initially make you feel alert and may be better enjoyed some hours before bedtime.

Regular use of alcohol or sleeping pills to aid sleep may require a careful assessment by a professional, to help with any underlying problems such as addiction or unresolved emotional issues. Such substances usually have a "knock out" effect rather than restoring natural patterns of sleep and dreaming.

A Few Final Words

So here we are, born onto this planet at a given time and setting. We are complex emotional beings, each unique and susceptible to changes in our environment. Given that we are composed predominantly of water and that the tides change with the moon, an awareness of our susceptibility and sensitivity to our physical and emotional environment is a key concept to keep in mind.

We hope life will offer us some amazing experiences but we know it will also challenge us in many different ways. At such times it is fundamental that we understand who we really are, accepting our underlying constitution and natural patterns of thinking, which we must both nurture but also confront, with love, compassion and where necessary, brutal honesty.

When our insecurities and fragile ego make it difficult to accept what we need to, it may be important to ask ourselves if we wish to live with emotional blocks and unresolved issues or to be free of such shackles and live with an open heart and mind.

Whatever choices we make in life, we must be clear about what we are doing and what emotional states are driving them.

Allowing ourselves to accept what is there does not have to mean reacting to it. Connecting with our breath at such times may help us to feel the nature of what we are feeling, whilst facilitating calmness. Think about where that irritability, anger or other emotion may be coming from. Sometimes it can be something as simple as being hungry, perhaps having had one coffee too many, or perhaps an underlying stressful situation playing on our mind.

We may find that our mind finds things to fit our physiological state. An example may be hunger resulting in irritation, with our mind recalling a memory that fits the emotion.

It is only by openly embracing a thought or feeling that we will be able to stand still and see it for what it is, rather than just react to it.

The same applies to certain habits we may develop. This could be eating something sweet that may not be so healthy, or the use of alcohol or recreational drugs. When such habits may be an occasional social and enjoyable pastime, they may be manageable and less likely to be harmful. But when they become an escape or habit with a degree of dependency, they will be harmful.

If we find ourselves in such a situation, let us be honest, explore what is happening and treat ourselves with love and kindness, even if we do not like who we have become and take steps to get back to who we are. This may require a deeper revaluation of our life, relationships, needs and wants.

In life we will hopefully be loved and nurtured by others, allowing us to develop a sense of worth. Some of us are not so lucky and may need to cultivate this by ourselves. Realising that love and forgiveness are prerequisites for our own growth and development, as well as for others for whom we care for, should act as a starting point. Without it positive change may be hindered by a misplaced sense of guilt.

We are not machines, rather complex physical, emotional beings, in some ways limited, but also capable of greatness.

Sometimes we end up in situations that may not be suitable for us. These could be a job, a relationship or even a home. We should feel nurtured, empowered and fulfilled by the things we immerse ourselves in. When you find it necessary, create a space for change and do not be afraid of where it will take you.

Clarity of mind will only come if we are honest about what may be driving us to remain in a situation and may require us to look at ourselves in a different manner. This may require a change in our self-image, who we think we really are or what we really need. At such times try and keep an open mind.

Practicing mindfulness, meditation and exercising can help clear the clutter. We are emotional and physical creatures and sometimes need to sweat and release the tension that stressors can cause by their physiological effects.

Do not underestimate the effect of stressors on your physiology. Having a physical form of release can be hugely beneficial to you. Try and develop such practices into a routine and you may find that what you need to do starts becoming clearer.

Be open to looking for different answers in different places. We are creatures conditioned by our environment, be it a culture or country we grew up in, perhaps a religious upbringing or certain values which we were presented. As we gain self-awareness with honesty, we may need to transcend our conditioning and understand that as an individual we may require a more open approach to our life, in order to feel fulfilled.

We are all going to die. Embrace that realisation and use it as a reminder not to waste time or energy with anything that is likely to prevent you from living a full life. There is no time to hang onto grudges; your heart and mind need to be open and free for what is important. Even if the emotional trauma we may have suffered requires time to process, be clear about our need to approach it and make peace with it. Invest time and energy in what feeds you, sustains you and loves you and hopefully you can live a life full of expression, growth and increasing fulfilment with an open heart and a calm mind.

References

It Goes Through The Heart

1. G. Rein, R. McCraty, et al., Effects of positive and negative emotions on salivary Ig. A. Journal For The Advancement Of Medicine 8, no.2 (1995): 87-105.

2. C. Kirschbaum, O.Wolf, et al., Stress and treatment-induced elevation of cortisol levels associated with impaired declarative memory in healthy adults. Life Sciences 58, no 17 (1996): 1475-1483. J.D. Bremner, Does stress damage the brain? Society Of Biological Psychiatry 45 (1999): 797-805.

3. R. Mc Craty, B. Barrios-Choplin, et al. The impact of a new emotional self-management program on stress, emotions, heart rate variability DHEA and cortisol. Integrative Physiological And Behavioral Science no.2, (1998): 151-170.

4. B. Barrios-Choplin, R. McCraty, et al., An Inner quality approach to reducing stress and improving physical and emotional well-being at work, Stress Medicine 13, no. 3 (1997): 193-201.

5. M.E.Bauer, Stress glucocorticoids and ageing of the immune system. Stress (2005) Mar, 8(1) 69-83.

The topic of cardiac coherence is covered in more detail in Dr David Servan-Schreiber's book: Healing Without Freud Or Prozac published by Rodale, 2004.

Mindful Meditation

1. S. Chaiopanont, Hypoglycaemic effect of sitting breathing meditation exercise on type II diabetes at Wat Khae Nok Primary Health Centre In Nonthaburi province. J Med Assoc Thai, 91(1), (2008): 93-98.

2. A. Hankey, CAM and Post Traumatic Stress Disorder. Evidence Based Complementary Alternative Medicine no.4 (2007): 131-132.

3. D. Oman, S. L. Shapiro, C.E. Thoresen, T.G. Plante, T. Flinders, Meditation lowers stress and supports forgiveness among college students. J Am Coll Health, 56(5), (2008): 569-578.

4. M.J. OH, R.L. Norris, S.M Bauer-Wu, Improved psychological functioning, reduction in stress symptoms, enhanced coping and well being in cancer patients. Integrated Cancer Therapy, 5(2), (2006): 98-108.

5. K.T. Deepak, S.K. Manchanda, M.C. Maheshwari, Meditation improves clinicoelectroencephalgraphic measure in drug resistant epileptics. Biofeedback Self Regulation 1994, Mar 19(1): 25-40

6. W. Sara, Lazer et al. Meditation experience is associated with increased cortical thickness. Neuroreport 2005, 28: 16(17): 1893-1897.

Dancing To The Ultradian Rhythm

This is based on the work of Ernest Lawrence Rossi Ph.D. and can be further explored in his book The 20 Minute Break, published by Tarcher, 1991, as well as through his website: www.ernestrossi.com

Maybe It's Something I Ate

Further details on the impact of foods on mood and well-being can be found in the following books on which this section is based: Mood Foods, The psych-nutrition guide, Ulysses Press (1995) by Dr. Michael Vayda. Looks at how nutrients and dietary deficiencies affect mood and function. Managing your mind through food, Grafton Books (1988) by Judith Wurtman, Ph.D. with Margaret Danbrot. Looks mostly at the effects of carbohydrates and proteins on mood.

1. F. Van der Eynde, P.C. Van Baelen, M. Potzky, K. Audenaert, Energy drink effects on cognitive performance. Dutch J Of Psych, 50(2008): 273-281

2. C.M. Beaven, W.G. Hopkins, K.T. Hansen, M.R. Wood, J.B.Cronin, T.E.Lowe, Dose response of caffeine on testosterone and cortisol responses to resistant exercise. Int J Sports Nutrition, 18(2), (2008): 131-141.

3. D.Graasi, C. Lippi, S. Necoziones ,G. Desideri, C.Ferri , Short term administration of dark chocolate is followed by a significant increase in insulin sensitivity and a decrease in blood pressure in a healthy person, Am J of Clinical Nutrition, 81, (2004): 611-614.

The information presented on Ayurveda can be found in most reputable books, such as those by Dr Vasant Lad or recognised course work.

Omega-3 Fatty Acids

1. S. Endres, R. Ghorbani, et al., The effect of dietary supplementation with n-3 polyunsaturated fatty acids on the synthesis of Interleukin-1 and Tumour Necrosis factor by Mononuclear cells, New England Journal Of Medicine 320, no.5 (1989): 265-271. A.P. Simoupolos, Omega-3 fatty acids in inflammation and autoimmune diseases, Journal Of American college Of Nutrition 21, no.6 (2002): 495-505.

2. D.O. Rudin, The dominant diseases of modernised society as omega-3 essential fatty acid deficiency syndrome, Medical Hypotheses 8, (1982), 17-47.

3. A.P. Simoupolos & N. Salem, Omega-3 fatty acids in eggs from free range fed chickens, New England Journal Of Medicine (1989), 1412.

The topic of omega-3 fatty acids is covered in more detail in Dr David Servan-Schreiber's book: Healing Without Freud Or Prozac published by Rodale, 2004.

Glossary

Amino acids: the building blocks of proteins.

Amygdala: part of the brain involved with mood, feeling, instinct and recent memory.

Antipyretic: having an action that reduces fever

Autonomic nervous system: part of the nervous system not consciously controlled e.g. beating of the heart, salivation and intestinal movement.

Ayurveda: a complementary health system originating from the Indian subcontinent.

Cardiac coherence: smooth heart rate variability.

Cardiac chaos: disjointed heart rate variability.

Circadian: having a twenty-four hour cycle.

Cortisol: a steroid hormone important for normal carbohydrate metabolism and stress response, which in excess can cause peptic ulcers, bone and muscle damage, hypertension, decreased immunity and can suppress growth in children.

Cyclic Adenosine Monophosphate (CAMP): known as part of the group of second messengers, which are chemicals released in response to e.g. a drug acting on a receptor. This then acts on a protein to cause a physiological effect.

Dehidroepiandosterone (DHEA): a steroid hormone precursor produced from cholesterol by the adrenal glands, gonads, fatty tissue, brain and skin.

Dopamine: a chemical having a role within the nervous system, often having a stimulating effect and a precursor of noradrenaline.

Doshas: the term for vata, pitta and kapha in Ayurvedic terminology, used to categorise most things.

Electroencephalogram (EEG): tracing recording electrical activity of the brain.

Endocrine: the endocrine system is an integrated system of small organs involving the release of hormones.

Free radicals: an unstable atom or molecule that may cause tissue damage.

Gastric acid: the acid released by the stomach to aid digestion.

Growth hormone: a hormone involved in growth, through protein synthesis, glucose production by the liver and fat breakdown. It is increased in response to fasting, stress and exercise.

Heart rate variability: the natural increase and decrease in heart rate by the opposing effects of the autonomic nervous system.

Immunoglobulin (Ig.): a protein acting as an antibody, i.e. acting against invading organisms or other complexes, foreign to the body.

Kapha: part of the classification system in Ayurveda, belonging to the doshas; it signifies certain qualities e.g. being dense, heavy or oily in nature.

Mucosal lining: moist covering of many tubular structures and cavities in the body, such as the sinuses and respiratory tract.

Neocortex: the outer matter of the brain.

Noradrenaline: a hormone and chemical, usually having a stimulating effect.

Neurotransmitter: a chemical substance released from nerve endings to transmit impulses to other nerves, glands or muscles.

Oxidative waste products: by-products of processes in the body requiring oxidation that are usually eliminated.

Parasympathetic: part of the autonomic nervous system that tends to e.g. aid digestion and slow heart rate.

Phenylalanine: an amino acid used to make proteins; it is easily converted to the amino acid tyrosine.

Pitta: part of the classification system in Ayurveda, belonging to the doshas; it signifies certain qualities e.g. heating and light.

Post traumatic stress disorder (PTSD): a psychiatric condition that may present after severe trauma and be marked by physical agitation, with flashbacks and nightmares of the events, as well as mood disturbance.

Prabhavya: Ayurvedic term to describe special effects of some foods that do not behave in a manner typical of their taste.

Sattva: Ayurvedic term to describe a calm, compassionate and clear mental state.

Sympathetic: the stimulating component of the autonomic nervous system that causes e.g. an increase in heart and respiratory rates.

Rajas: Ayurvedic term to describe an agitated, restless or irritable mental state.

Rasa: Ayurvedic term for taste.

Tamas: Ayurvedic term to describe a dull, stagnant mental state prone to depression.

Tryptophan: an amino acid that forms the chemical serotonin.

Tyramine: an amino acid, naturally found in cheese, which can have adrenaline like effects e.g. increasing blood pressure.

Tyrosine: an amino acid that forms the chemical dopamine and noradrenaline.

Ultradian: occurring more than once in 24 hours.

Vata: part of the classification system in Ayurveda, belonging to the doshas; it signifies certain qualities e.g. cold, permeable and rough.

Vipaka: Ayurvedic term for the latent effect of food having an increasing or reducing effect on the body, relating to metabolism.

Vipassana: meaning to see things as they really are. It is also the name of a meditation organisation.

Virya: Ayurvedic term for the initial thermal effect of food on the body.

NOTES

NOTES

NOTES

NOTES

NOTES

NOTES

NOTES